D1372838

MONOCLONAL ANTIBODIES

Diagnostic and Therapeutic Use
in Tumor and Transplantation

Edited by

Satya N. Chatterjee

PSG PUBLISHING COMPANY, INC.
LITTLETON, MASSACHUSETTS

Library of Congress Cataloging in Publication Data
Main entry under title:

Monoclonal antibodies.
  Based on papers presented at the International
Conference on Monoclonal Antibodies: Diagnostic and
Therapeutic Use in Tumor and Transplantation, held
Sept. 8–9, 1983, in San Francisco, Calif., and
organized by the University of California, Davis,
School of Medicine.
    Includes index.
    1. Antibodies, Monoclonal — Diagnostic use — Congresses.
2. Antibodies, Monoclonal — Therapeutic use — Congresses.
3. Tumors — Immunological aspects — Congresses.
4. Transplantation immunology — Congresses.
I. Chatterjee, Satya N.   II. International Conference
on Monoclonal Antibodies: Diagnostic and Therapeutic
Use in Tumor and Transplantation (1983   : San Francisco,
Calif.)   III. University of California, Davis.   School
of Medicine.   [DNLM: 1. Antibodies, Monoclonal —
diagnostic use — congresses.   2. Antibodies, Monoclonal —
therapeutic use — congresses.   3. Neoplasms — immunology —
congresses.   4. Transplantation Immunology — congresses.
QW 575 M7471 1983]
QR186.85.M659   616.07′93   84-26598
ISBN 0-88416-511-6

Published by:
PSG PUBLISHING COMPANY, INC.
545 Great Road
Littleton, Massachusetts 01460

International Standard Book Number: 0-88416-511-6

Library of Congress Catalog Card Number: 84-26598

To my wife, Patricia, for her help, interest and encouragement with monoclonal works.

Contributors*

Ronald Billing, PhD
Assistant Adjunct Professor
University of California,
  Los Angeles
Los Angeles, California

Karen G. Burnett, PhD
Senior Research Scientist
Hybritech, Inc.
San Diego, California

L. Chatenoud, MD
INSERM U 25
Hospital Necker
Paris, France

Satya N. Chatterjee, MD, FRCS,
  FACS
Professor of Surgery
University of California, Davis,
  School of Medicine
Davis, California

John Cicciarelli, PhD
Research Associate
Tissue Typing Laboratory
Department of Surgery
University of California,
  Los Angeles
Los Angeles, California

A. Benedict Cosimi, MD*
Department of Surgery
Massachusetts General Hospital
Boston, Massachusetts

Robert O. Dillman, MD, FACP
Assistant Professor of Medicine
Division of
  Hematology/Oncology
University of California,
  San Diego
San Diego, California

S. Ian Drew, MD, FRCP(C)
Department of Oncology
Wadsworth V.A. Hospital
University of California,
  Los Angeles
Los Angeles, California

W.F. Green*
Vanderbilt University
Nashville, Tennessee

John Hansen, MD*
Director, Histocompatibility
  Laboratory
Fred Hutchinson Cancer
  Research Center
Seattle, Washington

M. Jonker
Primate Center TNO
Rijswik, The Netherlands

R. Kurrle*
Research Laboratories of
  Behringwerke A.G.
Marburg, West Germany

---

*Those listed contributed to the Conference. Some did not submit their manuscripts, and they are identified with an asterisk after their names. Please note only first authors of presented papers are listed.

Lois Lampson*
Department of Anatomy
University of Pennsylvania
 Medical School
Philadelphia, Pennsylvania

Rosemonde Mandeville, MBChB,
 PhD
Professor, Immunology Research
 Center
Institut Armand–Frappier
Quebec, Canada

P.J. Martin*
Fred Hutchinson Cancer
 Research Center
Seattle, Washington

Richard Miller, MD*
Becton-Dickinson Monoclonal
 Center
Mountain View, California

J.L. Murray
The University of Texas System
 Cancer Center
M.D. Anderson Hospital
 and Tumor Institute
Houston, Texas

F. Pazderka, PhD
Senior Scientist
Division of Nephrology and
 Immunology
University of Alberta
Edmonton, Alberta, Canada

R.H. Raynor, MD
Division of Radiation Therapy
 and Oncology
Medical College of Virginia
Richmond, Virginia

Lana S. Rittmann, PhD
Senior Scientist
Hybritech, Inc.
San Diego, California

William E. Seaman, MD
Chief, Arthritis/Immunology
V.A. Medical Center
University of California,
 San Francisco
San Francisco, California

Zenon Steplewski, PhD*
Sidney Farber Cancer Research
 Institute
Boston, Massachusetts

Paul I. Terasaki, PhD
Professor of Surgery
University of California,
 Los Angeles
Los Angeles, California

Michael E. Trigg, MD
Department of Pediatrics
University of Wisconsin
Madison, Wisconsin

P. Vigeral, MD
INSERM U 25
Hôpital Necker
Paris, France

Contents

V. CANCER AND MONOCLONAL ANTIBODIES

Foreword

All academic readers are well aware of the discovery and development of monoclonal antibodies but few will have the in-depth knowledge or experience about their possible uses and limitations. The specificity and safety of this product is yet to be critically evaluated. No doubt monoclonal antibodies are powerful tools. It is the responsibility of the academic and research institutions to direct and guide all concerned so as to obtain the maximum benefit from this new technological advance. In this Conference we tried to discuss and share the latest information on this topic available from research centers throughout the world which is now incorporated in this volume. After one goes through this collection of papers, it will be obvious how difficult and complex the whole subject is, how little we know and how much is still to be discovered. The scope is unlimited.

The book is based on papers presented at the International Conference on Monoclonal Antibodies: Diagnostic and Therapeutic Use in Tumor and Transplantation, held on September 8–9, 1983 in San Francisco, California. It was organized by the University of California, Davis, School of Medicine. The organizing committee for the meeting was Dr. Satya N. Chatterjee (Chairman), Dr. Paul Terasaki, Dr. James Goodnight, Dr. John Hansen, Dr. William Seaman, and Dr. Ralph Reisfeld.

This book is meant for graduate students, for medical and nonmedical researchers in the field of immunology, oncology and organ transplantation, as well as for the newly developed industries in biogenetic research. Never before has a close and mutually respected cooperation like this existed between industry and science — a commercial union indeed. Each presenter was asked to submit a full length paper for publication. A few of them did not; hence only their abstracts appear in this book. Our apologies to them.

I would like to acknowledge my appreciation to the editorial staff of PSG Publishing Company, Inc. for their support and encouragement, especially to Dr. Frank Paparello, Publisher, and Bette J. Aaronson, Managing Editor. I thank everyone on the organizing committee for their help and suggestions, especially Dr. Paul Terasaki, without whose advice this symposium would not have been as successful. My thanks go to all the guest speakers and investigators who presented their work at the Conference. I hope you will enjoy the high quality of their work as much as I did.

Satya N. Chatterjee, MD

1   *T Lymphocyte Subsets in Renal Allograft Recipients*

F. Pazderka, V. Pazderka,
T. Kovithavongs, J.B. Dossetor

It has been shown repeatedly that subsets of immunoregulatory T cells in peripheral blood undergo considerable shifts after organ allotransplantation. However, the biological and clinical importance of these shifts still remains a matter of controversy. For example, it has been suggested that $T_H:T_{C/S}$ ratios in kidney allograft recipients may reflect nothing more than the efficacy of immunosuppressive treatment and are not directly related to immunologic effector function. This assumption has been contradicted by the observation of Ellis and co-workers[1] that specific anti-donor CML unresponsiveness is associated with periods of decreased $T_H:T_{C/S}$ cell ratios.

The clinical importance of $T_H:T_{C/S}$ cell ratio in immunological monitoring of kidney allograft recipients also remains controversial. After the original observation by Cosimi and co-workers[2] that patients with a stable ratio of above 1.3 are at greater risk of developing acute rejection compared to patients with low ratio, numerous deviations from that rule were reported, and the feasibility of T-subset ratio in prediction or confirmation of rejection was questioned.[3,4]

In part, this controversy can be attributed to technical reasons, especially difficulties in preparing pure lymphocyte suspension from a patient's blood sample, and evaluation of fluorescence in a sample containing lymphocytes at various stages of blastic transformation. In addition, the results are affected by different immunosuppressive regimens and the times when blood samples are drawn in the posttransplant period.

MATERIALS AND METHODS

Cells: Mononuclear cells were prepared from 14 ml heparinized peripheral blood by Ficoll-Hypaque density gradient centrifugation. Adherent cells were removed by plastic adherence technique. Lymphocytes were separated into T and B cells by AET-treated sheep red blood cell (SRBC) rosetting.[5]

Monoclonal antibodies: Aliquots of purified T lymphocytes were incubated for 30 minutes at 4C with the following monoclonal antibodies:

Leu-4 (marking all mature T cells), Leu-3a + b (helper/inducer subset), and Leu-2a (cytotoxic-suppressor subset). In several experiments, HLA-DR antibody was used as well to identify activated T cells. After thorough washing, antibody-treated cells were incubated with fluorescein-labeled goat anti-mouse IgG (TAGO, Burlingame, CA) following the procedure of Becton-Dickinson. Labeled cells were enumerated using fluorescent microscopy. At least 200 cells per sample were counted. Reproducibility of results obtained with such preparations was 0.93.

RESULTS

In our first set of experiments, we compared T-subset ratios in *long-term recipients* of allografts. Fifty-one transplant patients who had survived for two years or longer were studied in this group. All patients in this group were on immunosuppressive regimens of prednisone and azathioprine. The overall mean T-subset ratio was 1.97 ± 1.57, not different from normal controls: 1.93 ± 0.72. Patients were divided into groups according to kidney function.

Patients with good kidney function (below 200 μmol/L) had a mean $T_H:T_{C/S}$ ratio of 1.89×0.94. In patients with impaired but stabilized kidney function, the ratio was increased to 2.77 ± 3.49. However, a very wide range of variation in ratios was observed in this group, so that the differences between the two groups are not statistically significant. The ratio in the patients who have subsequently lost the transplant actually showed the lowest ratio (1.54 ± 0.55). Whether this signifies the decrease of immunological activity and cessation of chronic rejection, or is just a chance variation, it is difficult to say at the moment. Our observations in long-term recipients seem to be in agreement with the conclusions of Ellis and co-workers[1] and Colvin and co-workers[6] that in long-term grafts the correlation between $T_H:T_{C/S}$ ratio and risk of graft dysfunction does not apply.

In the second series of experiments, we studied the T-subset ratios in 38 *recently* transplanted patients less than one year after transplantation. The mean ratio per patient was calculated on the basis of 3–4 samples obtained at various intervals after surgery. The overall mean of T-cell subset ratio in this group was 2.17 ± 1.50. Data were analyzed separately for three subgroups: patients who had smooth posttransplant courses without rejection episodes; patients with one or more episodes of reversible rejection; and patients who subsequently underwent irreversible rejection. Patients with no rejection episodes had the lowest ratio (1.46 ± 1.43). In patients with reversible rejection, it was elevated to 2.52 ± 1.43 and with irreversible rejections, to 2.97 ± 1.15. The difference between the non-rejecting group and both groups with rejections was statistically significant (see Figure 1).

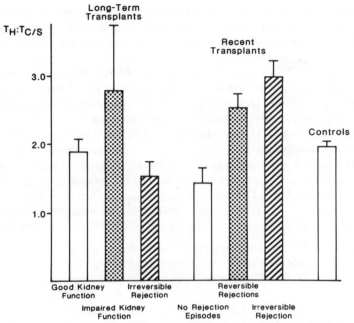

Figure 1 T_H:$T_{C/S}$ cell ratios in kidney allograft recipients and normal controls. Each bar represents mean T_H:$T_{C/S}$ cell ratio $\pm$ SE in a group of patients or controls. Differences between groups of long-term recipients are nonsignificant. Differences between nonrejecting group of recently transplanted patients and both groups with rejection was statistically significant ($p < 0.001$); difference between groups with reversible versus nonreversible rejections was not significant.

Thus, in recently transplanted patients, the correlation between the ratio and kidney function is obvious. However, the more important concern is the feasibility of enumeration of T-cell subsets in individual patients as a means of predicting the risk of graft rejection or detecting an ongoing rejection. This latter problem becomes increasingly important in patients on cyclosporine immunosuppression, since this drug is known to have nephrotoxic side effects. This means that when the increase in creatinine levels occurs, it may reflect either a rejection or cyclosporine toxicity. Obviously, the treatment in the two cases would differ considerably. To a certain extent, cyclosporine toxicity could be monitored by measuring serum cyclosporine levels, but individual variation in cyclosporine tolerance makes it very difficult to establish effective, yet safe doses for each patient. We have reasoned that if, indeed, an increase in T-subset ratio reflects activation of the patient's immune system, immunologic rejection should be accompanied by elevated ratios. In the case of cyclosporine toxicity, such elevation would not be expected. We have performed sequential T-subset determinations in 10 recently transplanted

4

patients. Blood samples were obtained before transplantation and then every week or, when possible, twice a week after surgery for two months. All patients were on cyclosporine (20 mg/kg) and alternate-day prednisone (1.5 mg/kg) treatment.

Figure 2 shows the posttransplant course of patient T.H., aged 15, whose end-stage renal disease (ESRD) was caused by membrano proliferative glomerulonephritis (MPGN). He had been on dialysis for half a year and had received nine transfusions. An increase in creatinine level from 90 to 150 μmol/L occurred starting on day 9 posttransplant. Levels of serum cyclosporine were within the safe limits, which we take to be 0.1 to 0.2 μg/ml (even though there may be considerable patient-to-patient variation). The increase in creatinine was accompanied by an increase in T-subset ratio from 2.4 to 4.8. This episode was interpreted as a rejection and the patient was treated with methylprednisolone, after which the creatinine leveled. The patient now has stable kidney function.

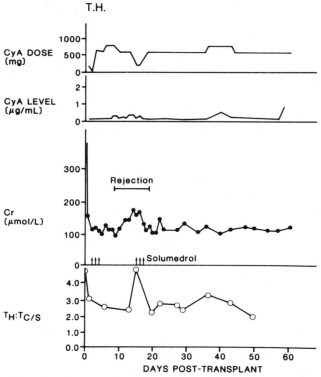

Figure 2 Posttransplant course of patient T.H., showing rejection episode accompanied by increase in $T_H:T_{C/S}$ ratio. CyA = cyclosporine, Cr = serum creatinine.

Figure 3 shows the posttransplant course of patient D.P., whose ESRD was due to Wegener's granulomatosis. He had been on dialysis for one year and was multitransfused. His serum creatinine started to rise on day 13 and reached the peak of 360 μmol/L on day 29. His serum cyclosporine levels were at that time close to 1 μg/ml. This was retrospectively interpreted as cyclosporine nephrotoxicity, not rejection. In this patient, the elevation in creatinine was not accompanied by a rise in T-subset ratio; it remained low during the whole observation time, never exceeding 0.7 μg/ml. No evidence of viral infection was found in this patient.

Figure 4 represents an example of an uneventful posttransplant course. Patient T.T., whose ESRD was due to MPGN, had been on dialysis for one week and was multitransfused (5 units) prior to transplantation. There were only slight fluctuations in his serum creatinine levels and T-subset ratio. There is no evidence of cyclosporine nephrotoxicity, although on several occasions his serum cyclosporine levels were as high as 0.6 μg/ml, nor was there evidence of rejection.

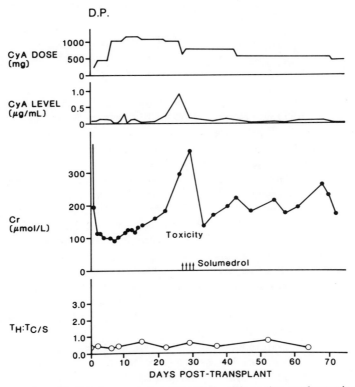

Figure 3 Posttransplant course of patient D.P., illustrating nephrotoxic effect of cyclosporine. Abbreviations: same as Figure 2.

6

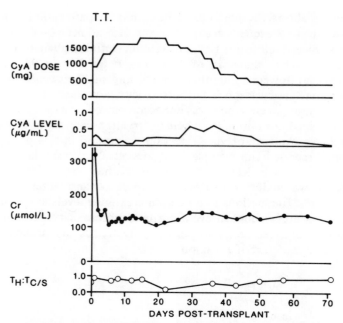

T.T.

Figure 4 Patient T.T., uncomplicated posttransplant course. Abbreviations: same as Figure 2.

Figure 5 shows the posttransplant course of the second transplant of D.O., whose ESRD was caused by type 1 diabetes mellitus. She received a kidney from a cadaveric donor mismatched for one HLA-B and one DR antigen. At first, she was treated with cyclosporine. After the initial drop of creatinine immediately after transplantation, her creatinine rose progressively to plateau at the level of 800–900 μmol/L, with some fluctuations despite several courses of methylprednisolone. The initial levels of serum cyclosporine were not indicative of nephrotoxicity. Later they reached the level of 0.7 μg/ml and stayed high for several days, after which it was assumed to be cyclosporine nephrotoxicity and she was switched to azathioprine. Kidney function, however, was not improved and on day 57 the patient started dialysis.

Throughout her posttransplant course, the ratio was high, never dropping below 2.2. Peak ratio was 5.9. It is interesting to note that her first graft was also rejected within two months. That course had also been accompanied by consistently high T-subset ratios.

Several investigators have pointed out that, when monitoring kidney allograft recipients on the basis of T-subset changes, it is important to relate the changes in the ratio to pretransplant levels. Therefore, we have determined pretransplant ratios in all recently transplanted patients. We find no correlation between posttransplant T-subset ratios, expressed as percentages of pretransplant levels, and subsequent kidney function. However, in retrospective analysis, we can generalize that patients with low pretransplant ratios had a more quiescent posttransplant course, with fewer rejections and lower creatinine values. It is possible that the pretransplant T-subset ratio may reflect immunological reactivity, and that a high pretransplant ratio may indicate a "high responder" to stimulation, either by previous transplant or blood transfusions.

We have examined the correlation of pretransplant ratios to the number of rejection episodes and the frequency of positive donor-specific lymphocyte mediated cytotoxicity (LMC) during the first four months after transplantation in 13 patients, using a T-subset ratio of 2.0 as a dividing line. As Table 1 shows, patients with a pretransplant ratio below 2.0 had a mean number of rejections of 0.2, whereas patients with a ratio over 2.0 had, on average, 1.4 rejections. The latter group also showed positive LMC at the time of clinical dysfunction in 10.3% of assays, whereas LMC was consistently negative in those low pretransplant ratios.

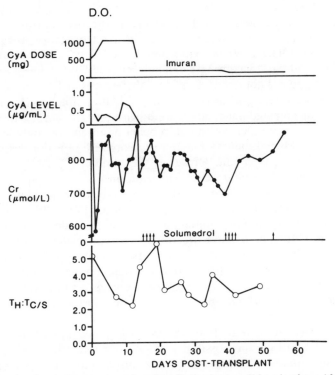

Figure 5 Posttransplant course of patient D.O., irreversible rejection. Abbreviations: same as Figure 2. Dx = dialysis.

8

Table 1
Effect of Pretransplant $T_H:T_{C/S}$ Ratio on Immunological Reactivity Post Transplant

$T_H:T_{C/S}$ Pretransplant	Number of Patients	Average Number of Rejection Episodes per Patient	% Positive LMC Assays in Relation to Phases of Clinical Dysfunction
< 2.0	5	0.2	0 (26)*
> 2.0	8	1.4	10.3 (39)*

*Number of assays for the group.

DISCUSSION

The value of T-subset determination as a means of immunological monitoring of kidney allograft recipients has been investigated in many transplant centers. Although a great degree of controversy is still present, the general consensus seems to be that a normal or high $T_H:T_{C/S}$ ratio is associated with an increased risk of rejection, whereas a low ratio signifies lower risk rejection.[1,2,7] This association is not found, as a rule, in long-term allograft recipients, which suggests that the mechanisms of graft acceptance in long-term recipients may be distinct from those operative during the immediate posttransplant period.[1]

Our findings concerning T-cell subsets in patients transplanted over two years ago did not reveal significant differences in T-cell ratio between long-term recipients grouped according to kidney function (Figure 1). In recently transplanted patients, on the other hand, the $T_H:T_{C/S}$ ratio is correlated to kidney function, the ratio being significantly lower in patients with stable kidney function than in recipients with rejection episodes and with irreversible rejection. However, the results of $T_H:T_{C/S}$ ratio determination should be interpreted with caution.

It has been pointed out that the ratio can be decreased by a superimposed infection, especially cytomegalovirus (CMV),[8] although it is not yet clear whether altered immunologic status precedes or follows viral infection. Colvin et al[6] have described CMV-associated glomerulopathy resulting in irreversible graft injury. In this group of patients, low ratios (below 1.0) were observed consistently. Thus, it appears that, in recently transplanted patients, $T_H:T_{C/S}$ ratio can serve as an indicator of the immunological status of a recipient, provided that the case is not complicated by viral infection.

Another factor that should be taken into account when evaluating the $T_H:T_{C/S}$ ratio is the possibility of selective redistribution of specific subpopulations: for example, sequestration of cytotoxic lymphocytes, at the onset of a rejection, from the circulation into the renal allograft. Analysis of lymphocytes obtained from kidney biopsy specimens, both in terms of T-subset ratios and their functional activity, would provide more direct information on the involvement of various T-lymphocyte subsets in the rejection process. This information would make the conclusions based on numerical balance of T-cell subsets in peripheral blood more meaningful. Studies of this nature are now being initiated in our laboratory.

In patients on cyclosporine, as mentioned above, it is very important to be able to distinguish between immunological rejection and cyclosporine nephrotoxicity. Cyclosporine blood levels are not completely adequate for this purpose.

Our data show that sequential measurement of T-subset ratio may, on occasion, allow differentiation between rejection and nephrotoxicity: an increase in serum creatinine levels due to toxicity is not accompanied by changes in T-subset ratios, whereas a marked increase in the ratio is noted in association with rejection episodes (Figures 2, 3 and 5). It must be emphasized that, for reliable results, blood samples must be obtained frequently and on a regular basis from the very beginning of the post-transplant period and continued for two to three months posttransplant.

Our studies have also shown a correlation between $T_H:T_{C/S}$ value pretransplant, and the number of rejection episodes and incidence of donor-specific cell-mediated reactivity (Table 1). No such correlation was found by Carter et al[3] in their comparison of numbers of patients with mean lymphocyte subpopulation values above and below pregraft means to incidence of rejection episodes. However, it is not only the shift in the ratio after transplantation compared to pretransplant value, but the absolute value of pretransplant ratio that affects the graft outcome. When, in our studies, we expressed posttransplant values as percentages of pretransplant level, no correlation with kidney function was found; when patients were grouped according to pretransplant ratio, the effect of that ratio became apparent.

We are aware, of course, that the number of patients followed is still too low to reach any firm conclusions. However, we intend to pursue this line of investigation by studying ratios in prospective recipients of kidneys from living related donors who are under the program of donor-specific blood transfusions. Sequential study of donor-specific and nonspecific reactivity in such patients should provide more information as to the value of pretransplant ratio in the prediction of graft outcome.

A large part of the controversy existing so far in this area can be explained by technical factors, as mentioned above. In addition, it becomes increasingly clear that T-cell subsets, as defined by presently available monoclonal antibodies, are functionally quite heterogeneous. For example, the so-called helper-inducer subset is now known to be composed of inducers of help, inducers of suppression, functional suppressors, and even cytotoxic effectors against DR antigens.[9,10] It seems reasonable to expect that, with the development of new monoclonal antibodies that allow dissection of T cells into subsets with more precisely defined functions, more effective immunological monitoring of organ allograft recipients will become possible.

ACKNOWLEDGMENTS

This work was supported by MRC of Canada. We wish to express our thanks to Ms. J. Clark for her excellent secretarial help.

REFERENCES

1. Ellis TM, Lee HM, Mohanakumar T: Alterations in human regulatory T lymphocyte subpopulations after renal allografting. *J Immunol* 1981;127:2199.
2. Cosimi AB, Colvin RB, Burton RC, et al: Monoclonal antibodies for immunologic monitoring and treatment in recipients of renal allografts. *N Engl J Med* 1981;305:308.
3. Carter NP, Cullen PR, Thompson JF, et al: Monitoring lymphocyte subpopulations in renal allograft recipients. *Transplant Proc* 1983;15:1157.
4. Guttmann RD, Poulsen RS: Fluorescence activated cell sorter analysis of lymphocyte subsets after renal transplantation. *Transplant Proc* 1983;15:1160.
5. Pellegrino MA, Ferrone S, Dierich MP, et al: Enhancement of sheep red blood cell-human lymphocyte rosette formation by the sulfhydryl compound 2 aminoethylisothicromium bromide. *Clin Immunol Immunopathol* 1975;3:324.
6. Colvin RB, Cosimi AB, Burton RC, et al: Circulating T-cell subsets in 72 renal allograft recipients: the OKT4+/OKT8+ cell ratio correlates with reversibility of graft injury and glomerulopathy. *Transplant Proc* 1983;15:1116.
7. Binkley WF, Valenzuela R, Braun WE, et al: Flow cytometry quantitation of peripheral blood (PB) T-cell subsets in human renal allograft recipients. *Transplant Proc* 1983;15:1163.
8. Carney WP, Rubin RH, Hoffman RA, et al: Analysis of T lymphocyte subsets in cytomegalovirus mononucleosis. *J Immunol* 1981;126:2114.
9. Thomas Y, Rogozinski L, Rothman P, et al: Further dissection of the functional heterogeneity within the OKT4+ and OKT8+ human T cell subsets. *J Clin Immunol* 1982;2(supp):85.
10. Meuer SC, Schlossman SF, Reinherz EL: Clonal analysis of human cytotoxic T lymphocytes: T4+ and T8+ effector T cells recognized products of different major histocompatibility complex regions. *Proc Natl Acad Sci USA* 1982;79:4395.

2 Phenotyping of Leukemia with Monoclonal Antibodies Using a Microcytotoxicity Test

R. Billing

Leukemia and lymphomas are heterogeneous hematopoietic malignancies corresponding to their various cellular origins. The subclassifications of these diseases have been shown to be important in the clinical diagnosis and choice of therapy. Previously this subclassification required several costly, sophisticated, individual, lengthy procedures such as histological straining; enzyme assays such as terminal deoxynucleotidyl transferase; detection of sheep erythrocyte receptors by E-rosette formation; surface membrane immunoglobulin determination by fluorescent binding assays and chromosomal markers. The availability of monoclonal antibodies against cell surface differentiation antigens has made possible a rapid and precise approach to leukemia and lymphoma phenotyping. Each subclass of leukemia has a unique set of cell membrane antigens that can be detected by monoclonal antibodies in a cytotoxicity test to phenotype leukemia. The antibodies plus positive and negative controls are predotted at appropriate dilutions on a 60- or 72-well tissue typing tray. The general specificities of the antibodies are as follows: T ALL, Pan T (T1, T11), Ia, SmIg positive cells, monocytes, myeloid cells, AML, blast cells, common ALL (gp26 and gp100). The microcytotoxic tray methodology allows for the addition of new antibodies as they become available. The pattern of reactivity of the lymphoproliferative cells against the panel of antibodies determines the subclass. Over 90% of random leukemias could be identified into the following subclasses: T ALL, B ALL, common ALL, T and B CLL, AML, promylocyte leukemia, CML blast crisis (lymphoid and myeloid types).

Lymphoproliferative diseases (leukemia and lymphoma) have been recognized since the early 19th century and are presently the seventh leading cause of death from cancer. Research in this area has been steadily accelerating since the early 1960s, stimulated by the availability of human leukemia cell lines in culture. At that time researchers began to standardize characterization, nomenclature and classification of the various forms of this disease in four main morphological subclasses: acute lymphocytic leukemia (ALL), acute myelocyte leukemia (AML), chronic lymphocytic leukemia (CLL), and chronic myelocytic leukemia (CML). In the 1970s, subclassification of these diseases has become more sophisticated and has

11

been shown to be important in the clinical diagnosis and choice of therapy.[1,2] Previously, this subclassification required several costly, sophisticated, individually, lengthy procedures such as histological staining; enzyme assays such as terminal deoxynucleotidyl transferase (TDT); detection of sheep erythrocyte receptors by E-rosette formation; and surface membrane immunoglobulin determination by fluorescent binding assays and chromosomal markers. The availability of monoclonal antibodies against cell surface differentiation antigens has presented a new approach to leukemia and lymphoma phenotyping[3-6] and also the identification of normal leukocyte subpopulations.[7,8]

The phenotyping of human leukemia and lymphoma cells has since become a fundamental, albeit expensive, research procedure. Labeled monoclonal antibodies in concert with fluorescent cell sorters are routine fixtures in large, well-funded research laboratories. However, the continual development of complement-fixing cytotoxic monoclonal antibodies now places this technological capability within reach of all. Using the proven microcytotoxic technology so well discussed in the literature and routinely used by tissue-typing laboratories all over the world, the researcher can phenotype human leukemic and lymphoma cells with a relatively inexpensive inverted phase microscope.

METHODS

Cell Preparation

1. Collect 10 ml of whole blood (or in the case of lymphoma, remove and process an appropriate node) into a 10 ml heparinized vacutainer tube containing 2 ml of RPMI tissue culture media with Hepes or equivalent and mix.

2. Centrifuge the tube for 10 minutes at 2000 rpm (733 g) in a Sorval GLC-2B or equivalent motor.

3. Using a Pasteur pipette, remove the buffycoat and mix with an equal volume of HBSS and layer a maximum 2 ml of the buffycoat-media mixture over 1.5 ml of Ficol Hypaque, the refractive index (RI) of which is 1.3545, contained in a 5 ml tube.

4. Centrifuge the tube for 10 minutes at 2000 rpm (733 g), again using a Sorval GLC-2B or equivalent rotor.

5. Using a Pasteur pipette, remove 1 ml of interface and place in a Fisher tube and spin at 4000 rpm in a Fisher or equivalent centrifuge. This will pellet out the leukemia and mononuclear cells.

6. Decant supernatant and lyse residual red blood cells with ammonium chloride; buffer if necessary.

7. Resuspend and rinse pellet twice in 1.0 ml HBSS or McCoy's media.

8. Count the leukemic and mononuclear cells on a hemocytometer and adjust count to 2×10^6 cells per ml.

Description of Leukemia
Phenotyping Tray (LPT)

One microliter of various monoclonal antibodies are added in triplicate to each well of a microcytotoxicity typing tray. Five to ten microliters of mineral oil are added to prevent evaporation. A potent anti-lymphocyte serum is added as a positive control and McCoy's medium as a negative control.

Cytotoxicity Test

1. Prepare a leukemic cell suspension of at least 90% purity and viability, adjust to 2×10^6 in HBSS, RPMI 1640 or McCoy's media.
2. Remove LPT from freezer, thaw, and allow to warm to room temperature.
3. Using a 50 μl syringe, add 1 μl of leukemic cell suspension (approximately 2000 leukemic cells) directly into the antiserum in the bottom of each test well.
4. Incubate the microtrays at room temperature (25 $\pm$ 3C) for 30 minutes.
5. Using a 50 μl or 250 microliter syringe, add 5 μl of rabbit complement to the test wells, directly mixing into the antiserum-leukemic cell mixture.
6. Incubate the microtrays at room temperature (25 $\pm$ 3C) for 60 minutes.
7. Using a 100 μl syringe, add 2 μl of filtered 5% aqueous eosin y to each test well (option: 1 microliter of 0.2% trypan blue may be used) and incubate at room temperature (25 $\pm$ 3C) for three to five minutes.
8. Using a 250 μl syringe, add 5 μl of filtered 37% neutralized formalin to each test well.
9. Place a 2×3 inch glass cover slide over the microtray and let the plates stand at room temperature for 15 minutes to allow the lymphocytes to settle. Observe the test microscopically at $150\times$ magnification under phase contrast illumination. The test must be read in 24 to 48 hours.

Dead cells (those with target antigen) absorb the dye and appear slightly enlarged and darkened, with distinct nuclear detail. Viable cells lack target antigen, exclude dye, appear slightly lighter and smaller in size compared to dead target cells.

After correcting for percentage of dead cells in negative control wells, the test is graded as follows:

% Dead Cells	Score	Interpretation
0	0	Unreadable
1–10	1	Negative
11–20	2	Borderline Positive
21–50	4	Weak Positive
51–80	6	Positive
81–100	8	Strong Positive

Results and Discussion

The four main morphological subtypes of leukemia have now been subclassified into eight major types that can be distinguished by cell surface antigens. The 11 monoclonal antibodies listed in Tables 1 and 2 react against a variety of different membrane antigens that are able in combination to identify these subclasses.

Tables 3–5 show the general reaction pattern observed with each cell type. The numbers of patients tested varied depending on the frequency of the disease. In common forms of leukemia, such as common ALL, AML, B CLL and chronic CML, more than 40 cases were phenotyped. In rare leukemias, such as T CLL, there were fewer than five cases.

There are some advantages and disadvantages of phenotyping by microcytotoxicity. The advantages of the LPT technology using the cytotoxic approach compared to fluorescent binding tests, such as fluores-

Table 1
Specificities of the Antibodies Used in the Phenotyping of Leukemia

Antibody	Specificity	Positive to	Negative to	Molecular Weight	References
CALL2	T ALL	T ALL	Non-T ALL leukemias normal blood cells monocytes	Nonprotein	9
CT2	Pan T	E rosette pos. cells	E rosette neg. cells	50K	10,11
T1	Pan T	T cells 50% CLL	Non-T cells	65K	12,13,14
CIA	Ia	Ia pos. cells	Ia neg. cells	28K, 35K	15
CB1	B cells	Surface Ig pos. cells	Surface Ig neg. cells	Nonprotein	16
CM1	Monocytes	Monocytes	Lymphocytes granulocytes ALL, CLL	Unknown	17

cent cell sorter analysis and flow cytometry, are as follows:

1. Fewer cells per test are used. The reaction of 11 antibodies in triplicate, plus positive and negative controls, can be observed using less than 100,000 cells. In most cases, fluorescent binding tests require 1×10^6 cells for one single antibody.

2. The tray technology requires no washing steps; as a result, the test is much simpler and faster to perform.

3. The reading of the tray is also simple and fast. Each reaction can be read in less than one second using an inexpensive inverted phase contrast microscope. Automated tray readers that will give the percentage of cytotoxicity in each well to within 1% are now available commercially. The reading of fluorescent binding tests requires expensive equipment and highly qualified operating personnel, or lengthy cell counting procedures using a fluorescent microscope. In our experience, because of the sophistication of flow cytometers, it is also a problem to maintain the equipment in regular working order.

Table 2
Specificities of the Antibodies Used in the Phenotyping of Leukemia

Antibody	Specificity	Positive to	Negative to	Molecular Weight of Antigenic Determinant	References
CG1	Granulocytes	Granulocytes CML-chronic phase, pro-myelocytic leukemia, leukemia	ALL, AML, CLL lymphocytes monocytes	107K, 140K	18
CAML	AML	AML	Normal blood cells ALL, CLL, CML	Unknown	19
CBL1	Blast cells	AML, ALL PHA blasts lymphoblastoid cell lines	CLL granulocytes lymphocytes	Nonprotein	20
CALL3 (J5)	CALLA	Common (c) ALL, CML blast crisis, lymphoid type	Normal blood cells AML, CLL	98K	21,22
CALL1	cALL platelets	cALL platelets CML blast crisis lymphoid type	Lymphocytes monocytes granulocytes	26K	23

Table 3
LPT Identification Pattern of Normal Blood Cells

Cells	CIA	CB2	CALL1	CALL3	CAML1	CMI	CBL1	CALL2	CT2	T1	CG1
B-lymphocytes	+	+	–	–	–	–	–	–	–	–	–
T-lymphocytes	–	–	–	–	–	–	–	–	+	+	–
Granulocytes	–	–	–	–	–	–	±	–	–	–	+
Monocytes	±	–	+	–	–	+	±	–	–	–	–
Platelets	–	–	+	–	–	–	–	–	–	–	–

Table 4
LPT Identification Pattern of Cell Lines

Cells	CIA	CB2	CALL1	CALL3	CAML1	CMI	CBL1	CALL2	CT2	T1	CG1
T Lines											
8402	–	–	–	–	–	–	+	+	–	+	–
HPBMLT	–	–	–	–	–	–	+	+	+	+	–
B Lines											
KM3	+	–	+	+	–	–	+	–	–	–	–
Daudi	+	+	–	–	–	–	+	–	–	–	–
Myeloid Lines											
U937	–	–	–	–	–	–	+	–	–	–	+
HL 60	–	–	–	–	–	–	+	–	–	–	+

Table 5
LPT Identification Pattern of Leukemia Cells

Cells	CIA	CB2	CALL1	CALL3	CAML1	CMI	CBL1	CALL2	CT2	T1	CG1
CALL	+	-	+	+	-	-	±	-	-	-	-
T ALL	-	-	-	-	-	-	+	+	+	+	-
B CLL	+	+	-	-	-	-	-	-	-	±	-
T CLL	-	-	-	-	-	-	-	-	+	+	-
AML	+	-	-	-	+	-	+	-	-	-	-
Lymphoid CML	±	-	+	+	-	-	±	-	-	-	-
Myeloid CML	±	-	-	-	-	-	+	-	-	-	-
Chronic CML	±	-	-	-	-	-	-	-	-	-	+
Sezary	-	-	-	-	-	-	+	-	+	+	-

18

There are two main precautions to consider when using the microcytotoxicity approach to leukemia phenotyping. If the cell population contains two or more major subtypes of cells, then the percentage of cells lysed may not be 100%. This would occur if the patient was in partial remission with 50% leukemia cells and 50% normal T lymphocytes in a mononuclear preparation. The phenotype of the leukemia can still be determined by, first, isolating the leukemic population by panning techniques, or by treatment with complement and anti-T-cell antibody (CT2) followed by percol density sedimentation. Alternatively, the presence of normal T cells could be taken into consideration in the reading of the tray. There will be partial lysis with T1 and CT2 due to normal T cells, and also partial killing in the wells in which the leukemia cells are killed.

Most patients at initial diagnosis have high leukemic cell counts in either the peripheral blood or bone marrow, and therefore this problem is not encountered in these cases.

The other problem to be aware of is that some leukemia cells are sensitive to certain sources of rabbit complement. Background problems can be avoided by using undiluted or diluted baby rabbit complement or B-cell complement (available from Pel-Freez).

Finally, some rare leukemias and lymphomas may have mixed phenotypes, eg, both T- and B-cell markers, and therefore they will not fit into any of the currently recognized subclasses.

REFERENCES

1. Billing RJ, Foon KA, Linker-Israeli M: The immunological classification of leukemia based on a rapid microtoxicity test. *Clin Exp Immunol* 1982; 49:142–148.
2. Cline JJ, Golde DW, Billing RJ, et al: Acute leukemia: Biology and treatment. *Ann Intern Med* 1979;91:785–773.
3. Sen L, Borella L: Clinical importance of lymphoblasts with T markers in childhood acute leukemia. *N Engl J Med* 1975;292:828–832.
4. Foon KA, Billing RJ, Terasaki PI, et al: Immunologic classification of acute lymphoblastic leukemia, implications for normal lymphoid differentiation. *Blood* 1980;56:1120–1126.
5. Foon KA, Schroff RW, Gale RP: Surface markers on leukemia and lymphoma cells: Recent advances. *Blood* 1982;60:1–19.
6. Kersey JH: Lymphoid progenitor cells and acute lymphoblastic leukemia: Studies with monoclonal antibodies. *J Clin Immunol* 1981;1:201–207.
7. Blackstock R, Humphrey GB: Cell surface markers in the characterization of leukemias. *Methods Cancer Res* 1982;19:51.
8. Billing RJ, Terasaki PI, Sugich L, et al: Detection of differentiation antigens by use of monoclonal antibodies. *J Immunol Methods* 1981;47:289–294.
9. Deng C, Chia J, Terasaki P, et al: Monoclonal antibody specific for human T acute lymphoblastic leukemia. *Lancet* 1982;1:10–11.
10. Kamoun M, Martin PJ, Hansen JA, et al: Identification of a human T lym-

phocyte surface protein associated with the E-rosette receptor. *J Exp Med* 1981;153:207–212.

11. Trigg ME, Billing RJ, Sodel PM, et al: Depletion of T cells from donor bone marrow with monoclonal antibody CT2 and complement for the prevention of graft versus host disease. Submitted for publication.

12. Billing RJ, Clark B, Terasaki PI: Characterization of three different human T cell membrane antigens, two being present on T lymphocyte subpopulations. *Hum Immunol* 1980;1:141–150.

13. Foon KA, Billing RJ, Terasaki PI: Dual B and T markers in acute and chronic lymphocytic leukemia. *Blood* 1980;55:16–20.

14. Kung PC, Goldstein G, Reinherz EK, et al: Monoclonal antibodies defining distinctive human T cell surface antigens. *Science* 1979;206:347–349.

15. Hocking W, Billing R, Foon K, et al: Human alveolar macrophages express DR antigens. *Blood* 1981;58:1041–1042.

16. Jephthah J, Terasaki PI, Hoffman R, et al: A cytotoxic monoclonal antibody detecting a novel B cell membrane antigen expressed predominantly on cells bearing surface membrane immunoglobulin. *Blood* 1984;63:319–325.

17. Billing RJ, Wells J, Suglich L, et al: A myeloid differentiation antigen detected by a monoclonal antibody: Characterization and presence on myeloid leukemia cells. Submitted for publication.

18. Civin CI, Mirro J, Banquerigo ML: My-1, a new myeloid-specific antigen identified by a mouse monoclonal antibody. *Blood* 1981;57:842–845.

19. Linker-Israeli M, Billing RJ, Foon KA, et al: Monoclonal antibodies reactive with acute myelogenous leukemia cells. *J Immunol* 1981;127:2473–2477.

20. Billing R, Wells J, Zettel D, et al: Monoclonal and meteroantibody reacting with different antigens common to human blast cells and monocytes. *Hybridoma* 1982;1:303–311.

21. Billing R, Minowada J, Cline M, et al: Acute lymphocytic leukemia-associated cell membrane antigen. *Cancer Inst* 1978;61:423–429.

22. Rita J, Pesando JM, Notis-McConarty J, et al: A monoclonal antibody to human acute lymphoblastic leukemia antigens. *Nature* 1980;283:583–585.

23. Deng CT, Terasaki PI, Iwaki Y, et al: A monoclonal antibody crossreactive with human platelets and common acute lymphocytic leukemia cells. *Blood* 1983;61:759–764.

3 *Monoclonal Antibody Intravenous Therapy in Lymphoproliferative Disorders*

R.O. Dillman

Hybridoma technology and large scale production of monoclonal antibodies (MCA) directed against tumor-associated antigens have rekindled investigational enthusiasm for passive antibody treatment of cancer. Animal studies have confirmed the therapeutic potential of MCA for in vivo antitumor therapy.[1,2] At the University of California at San Diego, we have been investigating murine monoclonal antibodies in cancer patients for three years. Table 1 summarizes our experience with monoclonal antibodies directed against three different tumor-associated antigens. A total of 42 patients have received 133 courses of these different antibodies over a dose range of 500 μg to 100 mg. One patient has been treated for over a year and a half.

This paper summarizes the results of our clinical trials with MCA T101. This is an IgG 2A murine monoclonal antibody directed against the 65–67 kilodalton (T65) antigen that is specific for T lymphocytes, thymocytes, and cells of chronic lymphocytic leukemia (CLL).[3] Reagent grade lots of T101 prepared according to Bureau of Biologic IND standards were provided by Hybritech, Inc., San Diego, CA, courtesy of Dr. Dennis Carlo and Dr. Jim Frincke. In fact, the simultaneous expression of surface immunoglobulin and T65 is virtually diagnostic of CLL or well-differentiated lymphatic lymphoma.[4,5] Inasmuch as most of this work has been published,[6,10] or is in press in a traditional scientific publication format, this paper is organized according to specific questions that have been addressed in these studies. Each section has its own methods, results and conclusions.

TOXICITY

There has been a great deal of concern regarding the potential for nonspecific, murine protein-induced hypersensitivity reactions and the potential for reactions associated with antibody binding to specific antigen. Table 2 summarizes the reactions we have seen associated with 133 infusions of MCAs in 42 different patients. Allergic reactions manifested by urticaria have been seen in 10–15% of the patients. The most common

21

reactions have been fever, sweats and chills, including shaking rigors. The latter have occurred only in situations in which the MCAs bind to a circulating target cell.[11] Thus, when there was less than a 25% decrease in the level of circulating target cells following a MCA infusion, no side effects were seen. However, when more than 25% of circulating cells were eliminated, there was a 50–50 chance of associated side effects. To date, all patients with CLL or cutaneous T cell lymphoma (CTCL) have experienced such side effects in association with treatment, while none of the melanoma patients have had such reactions. In one patient with CLL, who has been treated off and on for over one and one-half years, his typical side effects of fever, chills, and sweats were prevented by pretreatment with prednisone. Diphenhydramine has been used to relieve pruritus and urticaria, but has not, predictably, prevented recurrence of these complications. Only one patient has had a reaction approximating serum sickness. That individual noted the onset of urticaria ten days after a first infusion of antibody and three days after a second infusion. This was associated with arthralgias and a temperature of 99F, but otherwise no symptoms of true serum sickness.

A second factor that may be related to side effects is the rate of infusion. We have observed three severe reactions during the infusions: one episode of anaphylaxis;[9] an episode of hypotension with dyspnea;[9] and one episode of bronchospasm, which occurred in an asthmatic.[5] All three of these patients were receiving T101 at a rate of 0.67 to 1.0 mg/minute. It seems probable that the dyspnea/hypotension problem may be unique to the situation of rapid infusion of large quantities of antibody in the presence of large numbers of circulating target cells with secondary agglutination in the lungs and associated pulmonary edema.[9]

In summary, there appear to be at least two etiologies for the toxicities and side effects seen in association with intravenous infusions of MCAs. The first includes hypersensitivity reactions such as urticaria and true anaphylactoid reactions. The second, which includes fever and rigors and sometimes dyspnea and hypotension, seems to be related to the removal of circulating target cells, and is probably influenced by the target cell type, the rate of antibody administration, the rate of cell elimination and the total burden of circulating target cells.

BINDING TO TARGET CELLS

We have used direct and indirect immunofluoresence tests in analysis with the Ortho Cytofluorograf 50 H (Ortho, Westwood, MA) with 2100 H computer capabilities.[9,12] To measure in vivo binding of T101, peripheral blood mononuclear cells (PBMC) were incubated directly with a fluorescein-conjugated antimouse antibody. To determine whether cells were saturated in vivo, additional aliquots of PBMC were incubated with

Table 1
University of California, San Diego Monoclonal Antibody Trials

Disease	Antigen	Patients	Dose Range	Duration Therapy (days)
CLL	T65	4	1–100	1–510
CTCL	T65	6	2–100	28–210
Lymphoma	T65	2	3–10	1–28
RBC Aplasia	T65	2	2–50	1–60
Colon Ca	CEA	10*	0.5–6	1
Melanoma	p97	15**	1–10	1
	p240	3	10–50	1–2

*Includes 8 who received [111]IN-anti-CEA.
**All 15 received [111]IN-anti-p97.

Table 2
Toxicity/Side Effects of Monoclonal Antibody Infusions

Symptom or Sign	% of Courses (N = 133)	% of Patients (N = 42)
Fever (T $\geq$ 100°F)	16 (21)	45 (19)
Rigors/chilling	10 (13)	36 (15)
Urticaria/pruritus	10 (13)	12 (5)
Flushing	7 (9)	14 (6)
Emesis	2 (3)	5 (2)
Dyspnea/hypotension	<1 (1)	2 (1)
Bronchospasm	<1 (1)	2 (1)
Anaphylaxis	<1 (1)	2 (1)

additional T101 in vitro before being tested with the secondary reagent. Figure 1 illustrates the in vivo binding of T101 compared to the saturation of circulating target cells, ie, in vivo divided by in vitro. The data shown is for a patient with CLL who received five different treatments of T101 at doses of 10, 50 and 100 mg given as 24-hour infusions. The treatments were given weekly. Complete saturation would be evidenced by points around unity. As can be seen, a 10 mg dose was insufficient to saturate the greater than $100,000/\mu l$ number of target cells. However, at doses of 50 or 100 mg, saturation of circulating cells occurred, but declined over the 48 hours following completion of the infusion. In CTCL, with a much lower circulating target cell burden, complete saturation of cells was readily achieved and was sometimes sustained for over one week. Examination of bone marrow from patients with CLL, and skin biopsies from patients with CTCL, which were taken within a few hours of the start of a 24-hour infusion, demonstrated in vivo binding of T101 target cells at tissue sites as well.

24

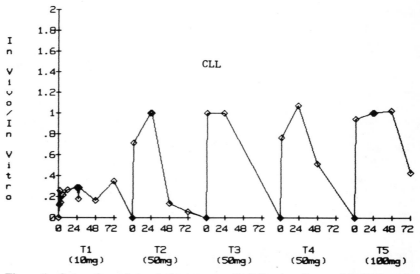

Figure 1 Saturation of circulating target cells following five weekly 24-hour infusions of T101 monoclonal antibody (dose). Values shown are for up to 72 hours after each infusion. "In vivo" refers to the proportion of cells coated by T101 in vivo. "In vitro" refers to the proportion of cells coated by T101 after incubation with saturating quantities of T101 in vitro. Fluorescein-conjugated antimouse antibodies in cytofluorographic analysis were used to determine the proportions.

BIOLOGICAL EFFECT OF IN VIVO BINDING

The binding of antibody to circulating target cells was associated with the rapid removal of such cells. Figure 2 summarizes the decreases in circulating cell levels that were seen in five patients who received 2-hour infusions of T101 as opposed to five who received 24-hour infusions. In both instances, there was a 60–80% reduction in circulating target cell number. This included patients with chronic lymphocytic leukemia who had initial lymphocyte counts of greater than 100,000 μl. Following completion of the 2-hour infusion, there were rapid increases in circulating target cell numbers back to the pretreatment level. During 24-hour infusions, the maximum decrease in circulating cells was evident at about two hours, then increased slightly, but remained markedly depressed throughout the 24-hour period of infusion. Once the infusion had ended, there was an increase in cell number toward baseline. Thus, it is evident that T101 infusions are associated with a decrease in circulating target cells, but this effect appears to persist only as long as an antibody is present, and is followed by a return of the cell number to pretreatment levels.

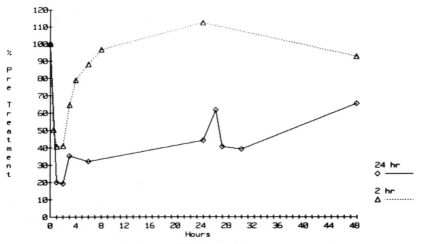

Figure 2 Decreases in circulating target cell numbers following either 2- or 24-hour infusions of T101 at doses sufficient to saturate target cells in vivo. Data shown are from five patients for each curve. Diagnoses included CLL and CTCL in both groups. In both instances, discontinuation of the infusion was associated with a gradual return of circulating target cell counts to pretreatment levels. Values shown were determined by dividing number of lymphocytes at each time point by the initial pretreatment lymphocyte count.

MECHANISM OF BIOLOGICAL EFFECT

The removal of circulating cells appears to be on the basis of opsonization with antibody and then removal in the reticuloendothelial (RE) system. We previously described an experiment in which ^{51}Cr-labeled autologous leukemia cells were reinfused into a patient 24 hours before he received an infusion of T101.[9] Immediately following the infusion of the autologous radio-labeled cells, there was a drop in counts per minute in the plasma as well as the peripheral blood. This presumably was due to the clearance of unbound chromium or chromium released from damaged cells, as well as the removal of cells that had been damaged in the in vitro incubation. In addition, there were very high counts present over the liver. Twenty-four hours later, following infusion of T101, there was again a drop in counts in the circulating cells in conjunction with an increase in counts over the liver and lung, as had occurred at the time of the initial infusion of the autologous cells. Subsequent studies have suggested that the spleen may be an even more significant site of removal of these opsonized cells; however, this study was performed in a patient who had undergone splenectomy.

At the bone marrow and tissue levels, it is not clear that any cytotoxic or cytolytic effect occurs in association with T101 binding. Neither

26

cell elimination nor attraction of mononuclear effector cells has been noted in samples of bone marrow, skin infiltrates or subcutaneous tumor nodules.

BIOAVAILABILITY AND PHARMACOKINETICS

A solid-phase enzyme-linked immunosorbent assay (ELISA) has been used to measure serum levels of immunoreactive T101.[5,13] Human T-cell leukemia cells were used as a capture reagent in this assay. Cells were then incubated with patient's sera and then with horseradish peroxidase-conjugated goat antimouse IgG (TAGO, Burlingame, CA). Substrate solution was then added and the OD 495 measurements taken on an automatic ELISA reader (Dynatech Instruments, Santa Monica, CA). Various solutions of purified T101 were used to create the standard curve used for quantitative measurements. Figure 3 illustrates the variations in serum T101 levels in a patient with CTCL who received four weekly 100 mg per 24-hour infusions of T101. With treatment 1, levels of over 300 ng/ml were achieved. One week later, this patient still had 92 ng/ml of immunoreactive T101 in his serum. Subsequent infusions of T101 were

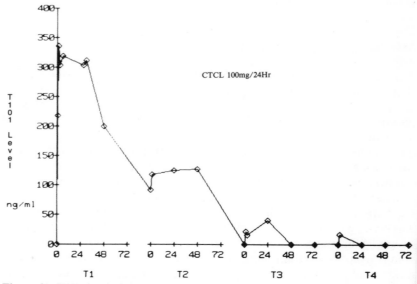

Figure 3 T101 levels following four weekly 24-hour infusions of 100 mg T101. Levels shown represent immunoreactive levels of T101 as determined by ELISA, and not merely antigenic mouse protein. At the time of the second treatment, T2 (seven days after T1), T101 levels persisted in association with antigenic modulation. The subsequent decreasing levels of T101 measured were due to the production of endogenous antimouse antibodies.

not associated with such high levels, apparently because of the production of antimouse antibodies. In patients with CLL, the ability to measure T101 levels was dependent on the dose of antibody given and the burden of circulating target cells. In general, for CLL lymphocyte counts of between 100,000 and 200,000/μl, T101 levels were undetectable at a 10 mg dose but were seen at the 50 and 100 mg doses. It was clear that a number of factors affected the T101 levels, including the presence or absence of antimouse antibodies and the kinetics of antigenic modulation. These are discussed below.

ANTIGENIC MODULATION

In vitro studies with T101 have shown that the T65 antigen is rapidly modulated in the presence of excess doses of T101.[14,15] This is true of cells from patients with CLL, CTCL and normal controls.[16] Our data confirmed that the same phenomenon occurs in vivo. One method of detecting modulation is to compare the expression of more than one marker that is characteristic for a given tumor cell phenotype. Thus, the percentage of CLL cells reactive with T101 is approximately the same as the proportion that are reactive with Ia antibody.[4] For cutaneous T-cell lymphoma, the percentage of cells reactive with T101 is the same as the percentage reacting with other pan T-cell antibodies, such as leu-4 or OKT3.[11] Thus, at any given point in time, the effects of modulation can be expressed using an index of the proportion of cells that bind T101 divided by the proportion of cells expressing either Ia or leu-4. When modulation is present, the ratio is less than 1.0. While mean or median intensity of fluorescence as measured by the Cytofluorograf is an even more sensitive measure of modulation,[9] this ratio method proves to correlate very well with such results.

Figure 4 illustrates the relation of modulation to cell saturation in a patient with CLL. Doses of 10 mg were insufficient to saturate his circulating cells and there was no evidence of antigenic modulation. However, at 100 mg per 24 hours, rapid saturation persisted for the duration of the infusion and then decreased sharply. In the meantime, by four hours into the infusion, there was clear evidence of antigenic modulation, which persisted throughout the infusion and then rapidly disappeared once the infusion had ended.

Antigenic modulation was seen in all patients who received prolonged infusions of antibody. In all cases, once the infusion had ended, the pretreatment phenotype was again expressed. In addition, when modulated cells were taken from patients and incubated in vitro in media of T101, there was also reexpression of the pretreatment phenotype. It appears that antigenic modulation is a dynamic phenomenon. The T65 antigen may act as a receptor and internalize the T101-T65 complex each time it is

28

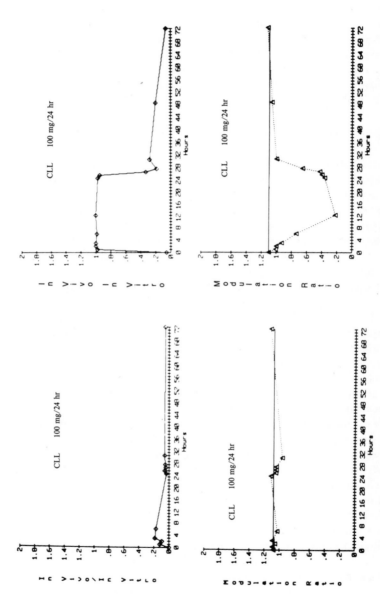

Figure 4 Correlation of cell saturation and antigenic modulation in a patient with CLL. The modulation ratio is the ratio of T101$^+$ cells to Ia$^+$ cells. Pretreatment, this ratio is close to unity inasmuch as most CLL cells are phenotypically sIg$^+$, T101$^+$ and Ia$^+$. A 10 mg T101 infusion was sufficient to saturate the large number of circulating CLL cells and no modulation was seen (left panels). However, at 100 mg (right panels), saturation occurred in vivo and persisted for the duration of the 24-hour infusion. Within two hours of starting the infusion, modulation was evident (decreasing T101$^+$/Ia$^+$ ratio). However, once the infusion was stopped and T101 serum levels

formed. During this period, additional T65 antigen is constantly expressed. However, as long as T101 is present in high concentrations, analysis at any given point in time will show only very small levels of the T65 antigen.

The phenomenon of antigenic modulation has significant implications with regard to the scheduling of antibody therapy. Prolonged infusions appear certain to induce modulation.[17] As long as cells are modulated, there will be insufficient antibody binding to the cell surface for cell removal in the RE system, or initiation of antibody-dependent, cell-mediated cytotoxicity at tissue levels. For passive antibody therapy, short infusions of a well-tolerated quantity of antibody are likely to be as efficacious as prolonged infusions. The therapeutic potential of a non-modulating antibody/antigen may be superior.

Antigenic modulation was also demonstrable at the tissue level. In patients with CLL and CTCL, in whom bone marrow or skin biopsies were obtained at the end of a 24-hour infusion, there was evidence of antigenic modulation, and no evidence that cells had been eliminated. This suggests that at the tissue level, antigenic modulation may occur too rapidly for effector cell-mediated cytotoxicity to occur.

ENDOGENOUS ANTIMOUSE ANTIBODIES

Because murine MCAs are a foreign protein, it was anticipated that antimouse antibody responses might be seen in patients who were not severly immunosuppressed. We have used a radioimmunoassay to ascertain whether antimouse antibody is present.[10] Patients were sampled prior to each weekly treatment. None of the four patients with CLL demonstrated antimouse antibodies, but four of six patients with CTCL developed antimouse antibodies within a few weeks of treatment. Figure 5 illustrates the relative change in antimouse levels in one patient with cutaneous T-cell lymphoma. That individual initially had no antimouse antibody levels, but by two to three weeks following his initial exposure to T101, he had exhibited a ten-fold increase in antimouse antibody levels. This was associated with neutralization of the T101 effect so that T101 levels were undetectable and neither saturation, cell removal, or modulation was detected. The fact that antimouse antibody levels have not been detected in patients with CLL probably reflects the immune deficiency associated with that disorder.

CLINICAL EFFICACY

Each patient was followed for up to two months for evidence of clinical response. No clinical benefit was seen in the four patients with CLL. In fact, in that disease, T101 seemed to have a stimulating effect

30

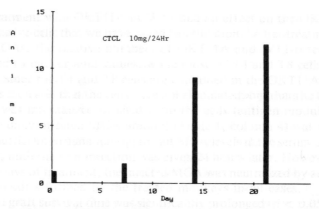

Figure 5 Antimouse antibodies as determined by radioimmunoassay in a patient receiving weekly infusions of T101. Values shown are an index obtained by dividing counts per minute minus background at each time point after an initial 10 mg T101 infusion by the pretreatment counts per minute minus background at later time points. Note the 10- to 12-fold increase in antimouse antibodies evident by 2–3 weeks after the initial treatment. This resulted in neutralization of the effects of subsequent 10 mg T101 infusions.

on the peripheral cell count. This was evident in one patient whose peripheral white count increased from 100 to 700,000 per mcl during the course of treatment. Subsequently, however, his white count fell to levels of less than 100,000 in association with a decrease in lymphadenopathy and splenomegaly. In CTCL, four of six patients had responses manifested by decreases in pruritus, scaling and erythema and an increased sense of well-being. The benefit in some of these patients was rather dramatic.[10] Unfortunately, all of these responses were sustained for only a few weeks at the most. In three of the four cases, the loss of clinical benefit was clearly associated with the production of antimouse antibodies that effectively neutralized T101.

CONCLUSIONS

We suggest the following conclusions and hypotheses based on our clinical studies with T101. The toxicity associated with the infusion of T101 antibody appears to be acceptable when slow infusion rates of less than 1 mg/minute are used. In a general sense, the allergic reactions to the mouse protein do not appear to be substantial. Delayed complications have been virtually nonexistent. One key observation is the association of side effects with the removal of circulating target cells. It is conceivable that the reactions associated with the elimination of circulating target cells might be more dramatic with different antibodies or antibodies directed to different antigens. In vivo target cell binding has been readily demonstrated with circulating cells and also takes place in bone marrow, skin lesions, lymph nodes and other sites of solid tumor. The biological effect of this binding to circulating cells is the opsonization and removal of circulating target cells in the RE system, especially the spleen. We have no evidence that complement is involved in the elimination of cells with the T101 antibody. At the tissue level, it is not clear that there is any biological effect other than antigenic modulation. In particular, there was no evidence of cell elimination or attraction of effector cells. The specificity of T101 appears to be quite good in terms of immunologic reactivity, but there is probably some nonspecific uptake in the liver. The bioavailability of any antibody will clearly depend on the dose administered, any burden of circulating target cells or circulating antigen, the overall antigen burden, the kinetics of antigenic modulation and the presence of antimouse antibodies. Antigenic modulation definitely does occur in vivo with T101 and suggests there may be no rationale for prolonged infusions of antibody. Endogenous antimouse antibodies were produced in several patients with CTCL but this did not take place in CLL. This difference probably is related to the difference in immunosuppression in these two disorders. It is conceivable that the antimouse response may be eliminated by desensitization procedures using higher doses of antibody. In terms of clinical efficacy, responses have been seen in CTCL, but these have been transient and limited by the production of antimouse antibodies. In CLL, we have seen no evidence of a substantial antitumor effect.

There are a variety of ways in which future investigation may proceed with monoclonal antibodies. First would be to look at the efficacy of combinations of different MCAs that react with different antigens. Nonmodulating antibodies/antigens might lead to more effective antitumor activity at the tissue level and thus a more significant clinical effect. Immunotoxins, immunoisotopes and immunochemotherapy conjugates may eliminate the problems with antigenic modulation and production of antimouse antibodies. Additional therapy to stimulate endogenous effector cell activity, or infusion of conjugates of effector cells and antibodies may result in an augmented clinical effect. Finally, production of satisfactory human-human monoclonal antibodies could theoretically circumvent many of the problems of antimouse antibody production or ineffective effector cell activity.

ACKNOWLEDGMENTS

The author acknowledges the collaboration of J.B. Dillman, D.L. Shawler, I. Royston, S. Wormsley, D. Frisman, M. Clutter, and P. Shragg in the conduct and analysis of the clinical studies summarized in this paper. The work was supported by NCI Contract NOI-CM-0744322, ACS JFCF Award #602, the Veterans Administration, Hybritech, Inc. and the UCSD

32

Cancer Center. The author thanks Kathleen Meyers for her technical assistance in the preparation of this manuscript.

REFERENCES

1. Foon KA, Bernhard MI, Oldham RK: Monoclonal antibody therapy: Assessment by animal tumor models. *J Biol Resp Mod* 1982;1:277–304.
2. Bernstein ID, Nowinski RC: Monoclonal antibody treatment of transplanted and spontaneous murine leukemia, in Mitchell MS, Oettgen HF (eds): *Hybridomas in Cancer Diagnosis and Treatment*, New York, Raven Press, 1982, p 97.
3. Royston I, Majda JA, Baird SM, et al: Human T cell antigens defined by monoclonal antibodies: The 65,000-dalton antigen of T cells (T65) is also found on chronic lymphocytic leukemia cells bearing surface immunoglobulin. *J Immunol* 1980;125:725–731.
4. Dillman RO, Beauregard JC, Lea JW, et al: Chronic lymphocyte leukemia and other chronic lymphoid proliferations: Surface marker phenotypes and clinical correlations. *J Clin Oncol* 1983;1:190–197.
5. Koziner B, Gebhard D, Denny T, et al: Characterization of B-cell type chronic lymphocytic leukemia cells by surface markers and monoclonal antibody. *Am J Med* 1982;73:802–807.
6. Dillman RO, Sobol RE, Collins H, et al: T101 monoclonal antibody therapy in chronic lymphocytic leukemia, in Mitchell MS, Oettegen HF (eds): *Hybridomas in the Diagnosis and Treatment of Cancer*. New York, Raven Press, 1982.
7. Dillman RO, Sobol RE, Royston I: Preliminary experiences with murine monoclonal antibody infusions in cancer patients, in Peeters H (ed): *Protides of the Biological Fluids*. New York, Pergamon Press, 1982, vol 29, pp 915–920.
8. Dillman RO, Beauregard JC, Shawler DL, et al: Results of early trials using murine monoclonal antibodies as anticancer therapy, in Peeters H (ed): *Protides of the Biological Fluids*. New York, Pergamon Press, 1983, vol 30, pp 353–358.
9. Dillman RO, Shawler DL, Sobol RE, et al.: Murine monoclonal antibody therapy in two patients with chronic lymphocytic leukemia. *Blood* 1982;59:1036–1045.
10. Dillman RO, Shawler DL, Dillman JB, et al: Therapy of chronic lymphocytic leukemia and cutaneous T-cell lymphoma with T101 monoclonal antibody. Submitted for publication.
11. Dillman RO, Beauregard JC, Halpern SE, et al: Association between disappearance of circulating target cells and toxicity during murine monoclonal antibody infusions. Washington, D.C. American Education for Clinical Research, May 2, 1983. *Clin Res* 1983;31:405A.
12. Wormsley SB, Collins ML, Royston I: Comparative density of the human T-cell antigen T65, BA-1 and Ia. *Blood* 1983;61:871–875.
13. Handley HH, Glassy MC, Cleveland P, et al: Development of a rapid micro-ELISA assay for screening hybridoma supernatants for murine monoclonal antibodies. *J Immunol Methods* 1982;54:291–296.
14. Shawler DL, Wormsley SB, Miceli MC, et al: In vitro and in vivo antigen modulation by antihuman T-cell murine monoclonal antibody T101. *Proc Fed Am Soc Exp Biol*.
15. Dillman RO, Shawler DL, Wormsely SB, et al: Modulation and/or im-

munoselection of human T-cell antigen related to dose and rate of murine monoclonal antibody infusions in man. *Clin Res* 1983;31:311A.

16. Haynes BF, Hensley LL, Jegasothy BV: Phenotypic characterization of skin-infiltrating T cells in cutaneous T-cell lymphoma: Comparison with benign cutaneous T-cell infiltrates. *Blood* 1982;60:463–473.
17. Dillman RO, Koziol JA: Mathematical modeling for monoclonal antibody therapy of leukemia. Proceedings of the 1983 University of California Berkeley Newman-Kiefer Conference. In Press.

4 Monoclonal Antibodies in Transplantation

S.N. Chatterjee

The last decade has witnessed enormous advances in our knowledge of the immune system. One such advance step was taken when Kohler and Milstein[1] described their technique of producing monoclonal antibodies (MCA). Monoclonal antibodies offer many distinct advantages over conventional antilymphocyte serum (ALS). In addition to the precise specificity for a single epitope on a complex antigen and potentially unlimited supply, hybridoma technology enables researchers to obtain pure antibodies with impure antigen preparations.[2] The transplanter's dream always had been to use an immunosuppressive agent that would work like the French exocet missile, selectively destroying the cells responsible for rejection of an allograft while doing no harm to other cells of the body. Utilization of monoclonal antibodies, a new approach to immunosuppression, may measure up to that test when used either alone or in combination with steroid and/or azathioprine.

PRODUCTION OF MONOCLONAL ANTIBODIES

The process starts with immunizing mice with suspensions of appropriate T-cell immunogens. Hybridomas are produced by the fusion of antibody-producing cells of the spleen from the sensitized mouse with a tumor cell line, eg, a myeloma that secretes immunoglobulin. The resultant hybridomas are distributed into multiple wells and the supernatant of wells tested by immunofluorescence on panels of T cells, thymocytes, and B cells. Hybridoma cultures showing specific reactivity for T-lineage cells are cloned and screened for the antibody to synthesize a specific monoclonal antibody. Because each clone is derived from a single cell, it will produce a homogeneous and chemically distinct antibody directed against a preselected, specific antigen. Further quantities of this antibody can then be continuously produced, either in culture or by injecting hybridoma cells into a syngenic mice, forming tumors and recovering MCA in the ascitic fluid of the tumor-bearing animal. Thus cells emerge that have a capability of producing monoclonal antibody forever — "immortalized," so to speak. The best hybridomas produce up to 100 μg of antibody pool in culture and 10 ml of antibody/ml in the serum or ascitic fluid of tumor-bearing mice.[3] The technique of monoclonal antibody production received a boost from the discovery of fluorescence-activated cell sorting (FACS). This technique allowed the sorting of cells bearing characteristic markers. Each cell is separated into a minute droplet, which is then deflected into separate containers depending on whether the cells had reacted with, and were thus coated with, a test fluorescinated antibody. Alternatively, indirect immunofluorescence has been used by direct ultraviolet (UV) reading in light microscopes. Less commonly, a cytotoxic assay has been used.[4]

PRESENTLY AVAILABLE MONOCLONAL ANTIBODIES TO CELL SURFACE ANTIGENS

Kung, working at Ortho Pharmaceuticals, produced various T-cell antigens, called OKT series (Ortho, Kung, T-cell). The antigens recognized by these antibodies are acquired and lost in a recognized sequence.[5] Main OKT antibodies are shown in Table 1 with the Leu series of Beckton-Dickinson shown in parentheses.

In normal adults, $73 \pm 7\%$ of mononuclear cells are T cells, $48 \pm 18\%$ are T-helper (T4), and $25 \pm 13\%$ are T-suppressor cells (T8). The helper/suppressor ratio is approximately 2:1.[6] The different subsets were summarized by Janossy and Prentice.[7] Circulating peripheral T cells are a mixture of T4 and T8 cells, which are also recognized by Pan T markers such as OKT3 and OKT1. In addition, there are T11 or E-rosetting cells that represent 50 to 80% of the natural killer cells. It is appropriate to mention here that double-labeled cells ($T4^+$, $T8^+$) are observed in limited proportions (less than 5%) in the peripheral blood of normal subjects but are present in high proportion in a number of pathological conditions, such as immunodeficiency syndrome, allograft recipients and cimetidine-treated patients.[4] These cells may be counted by double-labeling in light microscopy, taking advantage of the fact that OKT4 is of IgG2b class and OKT8 is of the IgG2a class.

WHAT CELLS ARE RESPONSIBLE FOR THE REJECTION PROCESS?

In the history of medicine cures have always been found once the cause of a diseased condition was known. Cure of allograft rejection has eluded us even though we think we know the cause. Clinicians all agree that the treatment of rejection and its attendant complications strongly affects the survival of the transplant recipients as well as the cost of transplantation.[8]

The cells responsible for rejection are macrophages and dendritic cells, which are responsible for initial recognition, processing, and presentation of the antigen; T cell helpers, effectors, and suppressors, which all play a role in humoral and cellular immune response;[9] and B-cells that mediate the antibody production. So in the past the rejection had been treated or prevented by the use of polyclonal response of antithymocyte globulin (ATG) with the attendant destruction of all T cells and increased risk of exposing the patient to neoplasia, fungal and viral infection. Even monoclonal antibody raised against Pan T cells (OKT3 or Leu-4) will have the same potential disadvantage. In fact, Cosimi reported a case of death following intravenous administration of OKT3 (B. Cosimi, personal communication, 1983). So we used the option thought to be safer—anti-B cell (anti-Ia) antibodies. Very recently, it has been suggested[10] that anti-Ia antibody reacts with Ia positive accessory cells to inhibit production of interleukin 1 (which in turn limits production of interleukin 2) and finally, T-cell proliferation. Our use of anti-Ia ended with death in four monkeys.[11] The cause of death was perhaps anaphylactic reaction: the lungs showed hemorrhage (Figure 1) while the lymph nodes showed selective depletion of B cells from germinal centers (Figure 2). Recently this

Table 1

Prothymocyte (immunoincompetent): OKT10
    (they lack 3,4,5,6,8,11)
Cortical thymocyte (immunoincompetent): OKT4, OKT5, OKT6, OKT8, OKT11
Medullary thymocyte (immunocompetent): OKT1 (Leu 1), OKT3 (Leu 4),
    OKT4 (Leu 3), OKT8 (Leu 2), OKT11 released into peripheral circulation
Helper T-cells: OKT1, OKT3, OKT4, (Leu 3), OKT 11 (Leu 5)
Suppressor T cells: OKT1, OKT3, OKT8 (Leu 2), OKT 11, (Leu 5)
Langerhans cells: OKT6

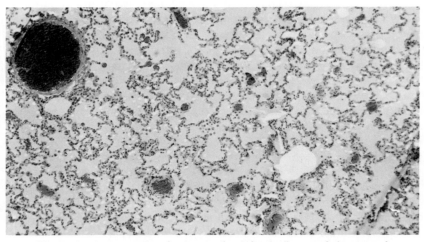

Figure 1   An example of a hemorrhage in the lungs of the animals.

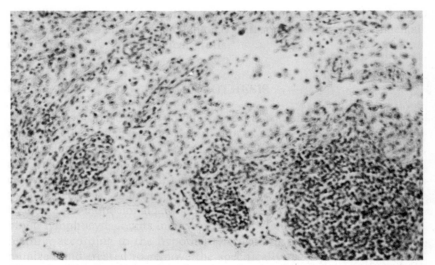

Figure 2 Histopathology of the lymph nodes showing selective depletion of B cells from germinal centers.

work was referred to by Marx in *Science*.[12] While attention was very correctly drawn to the danger of using Ia monoclonal antibody, the article failed to mention the second part of our study with antiblast monoclonal antibody.

Following the completion of Ia antibody studies, we decided to move on to the next most logically safe monoclonal antibody, ie, antiblast-antimonocyte antibody. The preparation and characteristics of this antibody have already been described.[13] Six rhesus monkeys treated with this antibody had skin graft survival of 16 to 22 days. No deaths or adverse side effects were seen in this group. Our study raised the exciting possibility that monoclonal reagents that react specifically with monocytes and macrophages have a significant margin of safety, and are useful perhaps because they remove or inactivate the monocytes and macrophages so that the T cells cannot be stimulated to act as helper cells or cytotoxic T cells. Treatment with this type of antibody will have the distinct advantage of leaving the normal T cells intact, so that the transplant recipient is not exposed unduly to develop malignancy, fungal or viral infection.

Clinical Work

Terasaki and his co-workers carried our work further in the sense that they used this reagent to treat clinical rejection episodes in eight cadaver and 11 DST-treated (one haplo-mismatch) living, related donors (LRD) (see Billing et al, this volume). Nine of the 11 living donor recipients were refractory to customary methylprednisolone therapy. Of the eight cadaveric recipients, six were refractory to methylprednisolone and four were, in fact, second rejections. The rejections were successfully reversed in 10 of the 11 LRD patients and seven of eight cadaver organ recipients. Most importantly, they confirmed in human beings our early experience of CBL1 on primates: These are safe reagents to use and have virtually no side effects. This observation alone should act as an encouragement to United States transplant centers to use this antibody. Mendez has used this and another MCA in Los Angeles and has found it to be somewhat beneficial (R. Mendez, personal communication, 1983).

Earlier Clinical Investigators

Cosimi was the first to use OKT3 to treat rejections.[14] His results and the results of the collaborative study of OKT3 are encouraging in the sense that almost 100% of the time the rejections were reversed. They did note side effects though and in one patient they proved to be fatal. There was another fatal case in Dallas involving the use of OKT3 (P. Peters, personal communication, 1983). The group working with OKT 11 at the Brigham Hospital[15] reported their results in 10 patients. They used the monoclonal antibody intravenously daily for 10 days. Reversals were noted in five of 10 patients. In an additional two patients, there might have been some role of MCA in the reversals. Three of their patients developed anti-mouse antibodies.

The French workers have used OKT3 as prophylactic immunosuppression as a single agent (5 mg/kg/day) in a prospective randomized study (see Vigeral et al, this volume). They reported no rejection episode for the first 13 days in all six patients treated with OKT3, who all needed steroids to treat acute rejection episodes after the first two weeks. Again, with the use of OKT3 these patients experienced fever, chills, and diarrhea, especially after the first injection. As early as one hour after the first OKT3 injection, a dramatic and concomitant decrease of T3, T4, and T8 cells was observed. $T3^+$ cells remained close to zero for up to 13 days post transplant, followed by a sudden rise and concomitant clinical rejection episode. Their other problem was noticeable immunogenicity when OKT3 was used alone. This problem was not seen by the Boston or Japanese group because they use OKT3 with conventional immunosuppression. Five of the six patients treated in the Necker Hospital series showed high levels of anti-OKT3 antibodies (IgG and IgM) (see Chatenoud et al, this volume). These antibodies completely neutralized the injected OKT3 and their appearance was invariably followed by clinical rejection. This is not an unexpected phenomenon and it could be prevented by the use of steroid and azathioprine. In four patients treated with conventional immunosuppression, the same group has shown that the antibody appearance could be delayed from day 9 to day 45.

AS A DIAGNOSTIC AID

Besides being a most useful tool as an antirejection drug and a possible tool for inducing immunotolerance, MCA can also be used in monitoring T-cell subsets. Cosimi found a highly significant correlation between kidney allograft rejection and OKT4/OKT8 ratio in peripheral blood.[14] Patients with a normal T4/T8 ratio had a higher incidence of rejection than those with a lower T4/T8 ratio in the first few months after transplantation. More recently, the same group observed that T4/T8 ratio correlates with the reversibility of a given rejection episode. Platt and his coworkers[15] reported that most infiltrating cells in a renal allograft rejection are OKT8 cells (cytotoxic cells), which play an important role in graft rejection. OKT8 cells in the future probably will be divided into cytotoxic (killer) and suppressor T-cell subpopulations. No clear marker-based separation of these two functional subsets has yet been reported in mouse or man.[4] It is not hard to predict that OKT4 also will be divided, based on markers, into functional subpopulations, ie, helper, inducer, and killer cells. At present, one does not know the percentage of suppressor cells in this OKT8 subset or the percentage of inducer cells in the OKT4 subset.

Disadvantages

1. *Immunogenicity of foreign IgG.* Following the use of mouse monoclonal antibody, 50% of patients will produce antibody against mouse IgG, primarily against mouse IgG determinants; but it can also be directed against the idiotype of mouse MCA, thus rendering further treatment futile. It could also produce antibody to anti-idiotypic antibody. This problem would be circumvented by: (a) using human monoclonal antibody, but here again this could also be rendered useless by anti-idiotypic response. Moreover, the major barrier to generating human antibodies is that man cannot be routinely immunized and bled just to provide such antibodies.[16] Secondly, only peripheral blood lymphocytes can be readily obtained for fusion and they are not as rich in fusible antibody forming cells as spleen or lymph nodes.[16] The other problem has been the lack of suitable human myeloma carrier lines to which normal antigen stimulated human B cells could be fused.[17] EBV-transformed lines may give us an answer; or it may be better to use recombinant DNA technology, with translation of isolated immunoglobulin genes either in a bacterial host cell or in a cell free system.[18] At present, hybridoma technology has had limited success in producing human MCA, although such hybrids have been reported.[19] (b) inducing tolerance of mouse IgG, or coupling the cytotoxic agent with the mouse MCA.

2. *Limited capacity to remove antibody-coated organ cells by opsonization in reticuloendthelia cells due to lack of effective macrophages and polymorphs.*

3. *Antigenic modulation*.

4. *Dilution*. Since the MCA must reach its site of action in appropriate concentrations to produce its optimum effects, several pharmacokinetic factors need to be considered. Parenteral administration will lead to the distribution of antibodies into various extracellular spaces, patterns of which may vary according to the class of antibody. IgG is naturally distributed extravascularly, whereas most IgM is located intravascularly, and IgA is located in seromucous secretions.

CONCLUSIONS

Products of hybridoma technology have opened a new horizon for us. In five years this new technology has reduced sophisticated tests like the Rosette test to insignificance, and is bringing in a new era in transplantation and tumor treatment. Little wonder that the lay press called monoclonal antibody "the smart bomb of biology."[20] One word of caution is in order here, and I will quote Brown,[18] "Due to the multispecific nature of antibody combining regions and homogeneity of MCA preparations, unwanted binding activity are likely to be observed and in man the binding may be totally unpredictable. Potential exists for derangements of the recipient's immune system which are likely to be more intense than the reaction seen in heterogeneous antisera." Nevertheless, the exciting potential is there to obtain many more monoclonal antibodies that will add a new dimension to the diagnosis and therapy of various human disorders. Thus it is with great expection that we view the 1980s in organ transplantation. Immunology now perhaps will be able to deliver rather than merely promising to deliver.

REFERENCES

1. Kohler G, Millstein G: Continuous cultures of fused cells secreting antibody of predefined specificity. *Nature* 1975;265:495-497.
2. Kung PC, Berger CL, Estabrook A, et al: Monoclonal antibodies for clinical investigation of human T-lymphocytes. *Int J Dermatol* 1983;22:67-74.
3. Diamond BA, Yelton DE, Schraff MD: Monoclonal antibodies: a new technology for producing serologic reagents. *N Engl J Med* 1981;304: 1344-1349.
4. Bach JF, Chatenoud L: The significance of T-cell subsets defined by monoclonal antibodies in human diseases. *Ann Immunol* 1982;133:131-136.
5. Reinherz EL, Kung PC, Goldstein G, et al: Discrete stages of human intrathymic differentiation: analysis of normal thymocytes and leukemic lymphoblasts of T cell lineage. *Proc Natl Acad Sci USA* 1980;77:1588-1592.
6. Chu AC: Monoclonal antibodies in dermatology. *J R Soc Med* 1983;76:1-4.
7. Janossy G, Prentice HG: T-cell subpopulation, monoclonal antibodies and their therapeutic applications. *Clin Haematol* 1982;11:631-660.
8. Russell PS: Monoclonal antibodies in renal transplantation. *Kidney Int* 1981;20:530-537.

9. Thomas F, Thomas J: Transplantation immunology, in Chatterjee, SN (ed): *Renal Transplantation: A Multidisciplinary Approach*. New York, Raven Press, 1980, p 1.
10. Silman SC, Roseberg JS, Feldman JD: Inhibition of interleukin synthesis and T-cell proliferation by a monoclonal anti-Ia antibody. *J Immunol* 1983;130:1236–1240.
11. Chatterjee SN, Billing R, Bernoco D, et al: Early evaluation of Ia monoclonal antibodies in prolonging nonhuman primate skin graft survival. *Proc Eur Dial Transplant Assoc* 1981;18:362–366.
12. Marx JL: Suppressing autoimmunity in mice. *Science* 1983;221:843–845.
13. Chatterjee SN, Billing R, Bernoco D: Early evaluation of anti-Ia and antiblast/monocyte monoclonal antibodies in prolonging non-human primate skin graft survival. *Hybridoma* 1983;1:369–377.
14. Cosimi AB, Colvin RB, Burton RC, et al: Use of monoclonal antibodies to T-cell subsets for immunological monitoring and treatment in recipients of renal allografts. *N Engl J Med* 1981;305:308.
15. Platt JL, La Bien TW, Michel AF: Interstitial mononuclear cell populations in renal graft rejection. *J Exp Med* 1982;15:17.
16. Diamond B, Scharff MD: Monoclonal antibodies. *JAMA* 1982;248:3165–3169.
17. Kohler G: Why hybridomas? *Hybridoma* 1981;1:1–3.
18. Brown NA: Prospects for human monoclonal antibodies: A critical perspective. *Yale J Bio Med* 1982;55:297–303.
19. Croce CM, Linnenbach A, Hall W, et al: Production of human hybridomas secreting antibodies to measles virus. *Nature* 1980;288:488–489.
20. Begley J, Hager M, Sandza R: Smart bombs of biology. *Newsweek* 1981; June 22:59–60.

Characterization of Human T-Cells and Their Subsets with Monoclonal Antibodies

R. Kurrle, W. Lang, E.J. Kanzy, T. Hofstaetter, F.R. Seiler

Therapeutical efficacy of monoclonal antibodies (MCA), and thereby an antibody-dependent elimination of a distinct cell population, is limited also by the rate of modulation of a given antigen. To overcome this effect it is desirable to use different MCA, characterizing T cells with identical functional properties simultaneously. We therefore analyzed in detail 8 human T-cell specific MCA. On the basis of the respective reactivity patterns, we could define three clusters of MCA characterizing three populations of T cells; mature T cells (Tpan); T-suppressor cells and T-helper cells. The assignment of these MCA to the respective clusters was determined by comparative analysis with well-known MCA (eg, from the OKT-series) by double labeling experiments, blocking- and cocapping experiments, and by analysis with cellsorter or antibody column separated cells.

The functional properties of MCA$^+$-cells were further analyzed in a PWM-induced Ig-synthesis system by co-cultivation of B cells with isolated MCA$^+$, MCA$^-$ cells, respectively (cellsorter/antibody-column-separation). The cytofluorometric analysis of the reactivity patterns of these MCA with human bone marrow indicate that at least the MCA against mature T cells should be suitable not only for organ transplantation but also to treat bone marrow for prevention of GvHD.

HLA-A,B,C Is Weakly Expressed on Neural Tissue and Tumors, but Can Be Induced on Neuronal Cell Lines by Interferon

L.A. Lampson

Monoclonal antibodies (MCAs) are of value, not only for identifying, classifying, and attacking tumor cells, but also for characterizing the tumor to better understand its behavior. Using MCAs to polymorphic and nonpolymorphic, conformational and sequential determinants, and both biochemical and microscopic assays, we have shown: (1) Neuroblastoma-derived cell lines express less than 1% of the HLA-A,B,C activity of glial, lymphoid, and many other cell types, per μg of extract protein. (2) The weak HLA-A,B,C expression is also a property of neuroblastoma tumor, and of neurons — and glia — in normal adult brain. (3) HLA-A,B,C can be induced on the neuroblastoma cell lines by interferon (IFN-γ). Implications: Weak HLA-A,B,C expression may protect transformed, infected, or damaged neurons from T cell-mediated surveillance. This may be a factor in the aggressive growth of neuroblastoma tumor, as well as in the immune response to infected neurons or neural transplants. Reagents that induce HLA-A,B,C may be of value in treating such tumors.

Lampson LA, et al: *J Immunol* 1983;130:2471–2478.
Funded by NIH #NS16552 and #CA14489.

Flow Cytometric Monitoring of Renal Allograft Recipients Receiving High-Dose or Low-Dose Steroid Therapy

W.F. Green, G.D. Niblack, H.K. Johnson, R.E. Richie, R.C. MacDonell, C. Ynares, M.B. Tallent

Renal transplant patients receiving high dose (60 mg/day) or low dose (30 mg/day) Prednisone in conjunction with ALS, were monitored for the first 12 weeks post transplant for changes in circulating lymphocyte populations. Both treatment groups underwent a rapid decline in total circulating T cells (T cell/mm^3) during the first week, reached a minimum in week 3–4 and then rose slowly to about 50% of the pretransplant value by week 12. The regulatory capacity, as measured by the helper to suppressor (T4/T8) ratio, was also observed to undergo a prompt inversion in both groups during the first week, continued to decline over the next 6 weeks and finally stabilized at about 0.50. Unlike the T cell/mm^3 data, the T4/T8 ratio did not tend to return toward normal; instead it remained inverted through the 12 weeks, and appears to remain so for several months. Thus, the quantitative and qualitative effects of the two therapies appear comparable. If, however, one examines the correlation of an increased T4/T8 ratio (≥ 1.20) with rejection a difference is observed in the two treatments. Patients on high dose steroids had a very high correlation of rejection with an increased T4/T8 ratio while those on low dose steroids did not. This suggests that there may actually be qualitative differences in the two therapies that allow the T4/T8 ratio to fluctuate more under low dose steroid treatment.

5 Human Monoclonal Antibodies to Breast Tumor Cells

K. G. Burnett, Y. Masuho, R. Hernandez, T. Maeda, M. P. King, J. Martinis

Within the last three years, clinical trials of mouse monoclonal antibodies for in vivo human tumor and transplantation therapy have become a reality, a fact to which this symposium attests. Prior to phase I and II trials, many clinicians and researchers were concerned that mouse monoclonal antibodies might be toxic to patients, as the foreign protein might elicit adverse immune reactions and, in the worst instance, anaphylactic shock. At this time, great interest was generated in producing human monoclonal antibodies reactive against tumor and other cell-surface antigens. It was reasoned that the human antibody protein might not activate the patient's immune defense as easily as the mouse protein. In reality, as documented by the reports of this symposium, mouse antibody toxicity is highly individual, depending both on the antibody, the antigen, and the specific patient. While some antibodies elicit various toxic reactions, particularly during first dose administration, other antibodies have been safely administered in multiple doses over the past several years (see Dillman, this volume). Selection of appropriate antibodies and antigen targets, as well as modification of treatment protocol and some adjuvant therapy, has in most cases eliminated any significant mouse-antibody toxicity.

Rather than toxicity, the major problem with mouse monoclonal antibody in tumor immunotherapy appears to be a gradual decline in efficacy during multiple dose regimens. This decrease in clinical response has been correlated with the development of antimouse antibodies that rapidly clear the therapeutic agent from the circulation (see Dillman; Jonker et al; and Chatenoud et al, this volume). There are three immediately evident solutions to this problem. First, treatment regimens might be modified to require a single dose of antibody. Second, it may be possible to suppress the patient's immune system during immunotherapy using drugs such as azathioprine or corticosteroids. Third, it might be possible to use a human antibody, which should not as easily elicit the patient's immune response.

47

The first solution, single dose therapy, might be feasible when using antibody-drug or antibody-toxin conjugates expected to have drastic and immediate effect on target cells. However, unless the initial treatment is one hundred percent effective, further doses of the antibody-based pharmaceutical would have to be administered either immediately or after a recurrence of the illness. In addition, only one illness could be addressed with the mouse antibody technique. Logically, we must find a means of administering multiple dose schedules of monoclonal antibodies.

The second means to avoid antimouse response is to use drugs that suppress the patient's immune system. Such immune-suppressive therapy is currently being used in various ways — for example, in the treatment of graft rejection, as discussed by others in this symposium. However, in the case of tumor patients whose immune systems are already compromised as a result of the disease and/or radiation and chemotherapy, it is not particularly desirable to use immune suppressive drugs. Vestiges of the immune system that remain intact should be bolstered, not destroyed, by tumor immunotherapy.

Therefore, the third alternative, replacing mouse antibodies with human antibodies, continues to be of considerable interest in tumor immunotherapy. We have been developing human monoclonal antibodies that bind to tumor associated antigens because we feel they might provide the ideal solution to the problem of inactivation of mouse antibody-based pharmaceuticals by the patient's immune response. This, of course, is not to ignore the possible problem of anti-idiotype antibodies. The extent of anti-idiotype response is difficult to measure and techniques are now being developed to assay this fraction of the human antimouse immune response. When human monoclonal antibodies are tested in humans it will be critical to monitor the extent of immunological recognition and the complications that might arise from it.

In addition to our interest in human monoclonal antibodies as therapeutic tools, we also feel that human antibodies might provide a distinct advantage in identifying tumor-associated antigens. A major difficulty in identifying human tumor antigens by conventional mouse or rat hybridoma technology is that a xenogenetically immunized animal does not distinguish tumor and normal antigens on human tumor cells used as an immunogen. Screening hundreds or thousands of these mouse or rat antibodies is tedious and does not easily yield antibodies to tumor antigens, which may be in low concentrations or relatively nonimmunogenic.

However, the autologous immunization of a patient by his own tumor should produce a relatively restricted range of antibody specificities, with a high percentage of the patient's antibodies directed against unique antigens appearing on the tumor tissue. Immortalization and screening of these human antibodies should help to identify rare tumor antigens and provide a means for isolating those antigens for various purposes (including generating immunogen for producing mouse monoclonal antibodies to tumor antigens).

And, of course, by immortalizing individual human lymphocytes and studying the spectrum of human monoclonal antibodies so produced, we may learn something about tumor immunology. The way in which humans respond to their own tumors and/or foreign proteins still remains an area of basic research.

While there is great interest in the area of human monoclonal antibodies, progress has been difficult. Major problems exist in three critical areas. First, it is difficult to obtain human lymphocytes producing antibodies of defined antigen specificity. It is even more difficult to find a specific antibody with the characteristics necessary for a good pharmaceutical reagent. For example, many hundreds of mouse monoclonal antibodies with appropriate specificity must be tested to find the one tailormade for a given in vitro or in vivo application. In most instances, it is not ethically justified to immunize hundreds of humans with antigens of interest and obtain spleens at optimal times after immunizations, as can be done in producing mouse or rat monoclonal antibodies. Second, specific antibody-producing lymphocytes must be established in long-term culture in order to clone out and produce a large enough quantity of each antibody to identify those of interest. Third, large amounts of pharmaceutical grade material must be produced in order to test human antibodies in vivo in animal models and in humans.

Highlighting these areas of primary interest, this paper will describe our progress in the area of producing human monoclonal antibodies directed against human tumor-associated antigens, with the aim of obtaining antibodies with the necessary specificity and physico-chemical characteristics and in the quantities that will be necessary for in vivo therapeutic application.

IMMORTALIZATION

As will be discussed later, the sources of immune lymphocytes of desired specificities is limited. Therefore, development work in human monoclonal antibody production must concentrate on optimizing yields of useful monoclonal antibodies from any given lymphocyte population. We have made a significant effort in the area of lymphocyte immortalization. We have looked for a means of growing human lymphocytes that yields a high percentage of useful clonal cultures that grow rapidly, make large amounts of antibody, are stable in long-term culture, and are a safe source of antibody for in vivo human use.

Three techniques have been considered as potential means for immortalizing human antibody-producing lymphocytes: in vitro culture of primary B cells, Epstein-Barr virus (EBV) transformation, and hybridoma production. Procedures for long-term culture of primary lymphocytes are currently being developed and have reached some sophistication for T cells.[1] With the recent flurry of research reports on B cell growth factor,[2-4,5] it is likely that within a few years it will be practical to grow and subclone antibody-producing B lymphocytes of interest. Such procedures may yield fast-growing, easily cloned B-cell populations with high antibody production rates. But at this time, our level of understanding of B cell activation, proliferation, and antibody secretion rate is insufficient to warrant selection of this immortalization procedure for the immediate goal of producing antigen-specific human monoclonal antibodies.

On the other hand, EBV transformation has now been used in numerous laboratories to produce human monoclonal antibodies of many different specificities. This technique has many advantages; particularly useful is the high transformation frequency routinely obtained. Some workers initially reported problems with instability and low antibody yields from transformed and subcloned lymphocyte cultures. Recent reports have been more encouraging. For example, Rosen et al[6] have produced human monoclonal antibodies to a genus-specific chlamydial antigen; Winger et al[7] have demonstrated production of human monoclonal antibodies to chicken red blood cells (RBC), neuraminidase-treated human RBCs, DNA-coated sheep RBC, and sea urchin sperm; Monjour et al[8] have described production of human monoclonal antibodies to *Plasmodium falciparum*; and Watson et al[9] have produced human monoclonal antibodies to melanoma antigens. In all of these reports, EBV transformation was used as the means of immortalizing an antigen-enriched human lymphocyte population producing the antibody of desired specificity. Obviously, EBV transformation has great potential in human monoclonal antibody production. However, an important concern is the presence of viral contaminants in the lymphocyte cultures. It may be difficult to justify the use of material potentially contaminated with a transforming agent for treatment of human patients.

The third technique for lymphocyte immortalization, hybridoma formation, might provide a means of circumventing the EBV problem. Mouse monoclonal antibodies produced by mouse hybridomas are not contaminated with EBV and have been approved and used safely in humans. The procedures for producing human hybridomas are much less well defined, but the mouse system presents us with a model of feasibility. By hybridoma technology it should be possible to generate human monoclonal antibodies that are not associated with EBV-transformed cells. We have therefore chosen to use hybridoma technology to produce human monoclonal antibodies, because it presents the best immediate prospect for making large amounts of antibody that might be approved for use in humans.

HYBRIDOMA PRODUCTION

The first and most critical component to hybridoma production is the choice of the most suitable lymphoid partner for fusion to immune lymphocytes. It took at least five years of research effort in numerous laboratories to make the mouse hybridoma system work. It was, in large part, the choice of myeloma P3x63 that made Kohler and Milstein's experiments successful.[10] Even today, the majority of mouse hybridomas are made with cell lines derived from the same P3x63 myeloma mutant. The search for a human equivalent to the mouse myeloma P3x63 has been difficult and full of half successes.

Very few true human myelomas have been established in culture. Of these, only a small number have been genetically engineered to be used like the mouse myelomas in the hypoxanthine-aminopterin-thymidine (HAT) selective system.[11] Olsson and Kaplan[12] first reported success in producing human hybridomas with the human myeloma mutant SKO 007. This cell line has been less successful in other laboratories.[13] Other HAT-sensitive mutants have been derived from the human myeloma lines RPMI8226[14] and U266,[15] which have been of some limited success in human hybridoma production.

Many laboratories have tried to develop human lymphoblastoid cell lines as fusion partners. Although many such cell lines exist, only a subset have been selected to HAT-sensitivity. Fusion success with these lymphoblastoid mutants is variable. Recently, several groups have performed comparisons among the human lines with respect to clone production, stability, and immunoglobulin secretion rates.[13,15] In most laboratories several problems plague the human hybridoma system whether myeloma or lymphoblastoid fusion partners are used: low and unreproducible yield of hybrids, low Ig secretion rates, slow growth rates, limited success in large-scale antibody production techniques. In addition, for all hybrids made with lymphoblastoid cell lines there is the added complication of EBV contamination.

A second avenue for producing human Ig-secreting hybridomas is to fuse human lymphocytes to the highly successful mouse myeloma lines. The first reports of such mouse-human hybridomas producing specific human antibody[16,17] confirmed what had been expected. Interspecific hybrids of rodent and human cells rapidly segregated human chromosomes. Therefore, when mouse-human hybridomas producing human Ig of a desired specificity were identified, the human chromosome coding for that Ig molecule would be lost and the cells would soon stop secreting the human antibody. However, these reports indicated good fusibility of mouse myelomas to human lymphocytes.

Therefore, in testing the feasibility of immortalizing human lymphocytes by hybridoma technology, we surveyed several human lymphoid

52

tumor lines and several mouse myeloma lines. In each instance, we measured fusibility, growth rates, yield of Ig-producing hybridomas, Ig secretion rates, and stability. The results have convinced us that the mouse myeloma line P3/HT is the lymphoid line of choice for producing antigen-specific human monoclonal antibodies.

FUSION OF MOUSE MYELOMAS WITH HUMAN LYMPHOCYTES

The eight lymphoid lines tested as fusion partners for human lymphocytes are listed in Table 1. We fused these lines to human lymphocytes from peripheral blood (pbls), tonsil, spleen, and lymph nodes. The results of these fusions are presented in Table 2. There are two immediately obvious points to be made from this fusion survey. First, pbls are the least fusbile of the lymphocyte sources. This is not surprising, as antigen-activated lymphocytes show the highest fusion frequency, and these cells appear only briefly in the circulation after antigen stimulation. Second, pbl fusibility is highly variable, depending on the lymphocyte donor. By using lymphocytes from several donors one can obtain a general idea of fusion success for a given lymphoid tumor line. However, the only truly effective comparison of fusibility among several cell lines must use the same lymphocyte pool. Day-to-day variability in fusibility of the lymphoid tumor line itself is also important and can drastically alter fusion outcome. Care must be taken to handle the cell lines identically before each fusion.

In our hands, the most fusible human line is 729/HT, a subline of 729-6 derived by Lever et al[18] from WIL-2. This line, in many instances,

Table 1
Lymphoid Lines Surveyed

Name	Species Origin	Developer	Parent Line	Ig Production	Cell Type
729-6/HT	Human	Seegmiller	729-6	IgM, $\varkappa$	EBV$^+$ Lymphoblastoid
ARH077 Az	Human	Royston	ARH077	IgGγ_1,$\varkappa$	EBV$^+$ Lymphoblastoid
GM607.11	Human	Hybritech	GM607	IgM,$\varkappa$	EBV$^+$ Lymphoblastoid
GM4672	Human	Croce	GM1500	IgGγ_2,$\varkappa$	EBV$^+$ Lymphoblastoid
NS-1	Mouse	Milstein	P3x63Ag8	$\varkappa$	Plasmacytoma
SP2/0	Mouse	Schulman	NS-1	None	Hybridoma
P3/HT	Mouse	Hybritech	P3x63Ag8	None	Plasmacytoma

Table 2
Fusibility of Human and Mouse Lymphoid Lines with Human Lymphocytes

Lymphocyte Source	Lymphoid Cell	No. Fusions	Total No. Lymphocytes	No. Donors	Total No. Clones	Range of Fusion Frequencies	No. Clones/10^6 Lymphocytes (Σ)
Peripheral Blood	729/HT	41	92×10^7	10	22	$<0.5\text{-}2.0 \times 10^{-7}$	0.02
	ARH077	9	20×10^7	4	0	$<0.1 \times 10^{-7}$	0
	GM607.11	19	65×10^7	8	6	$<0.1\text{-}2.0 \times 10^{-7}$	0.01
	GM4672	3	3.0×10^7	1	1	$<0.3\text{-}1.0 \times 10^{-7}$	0.03
	NS-1	9	15×10^7	4	98	$<2.0\text{-}30 \times 10^{-7}$	0.7
	SP2/0	69	85×10^7	20	2143	$<0.2\text{-}200 \times 10^{-7}$	2.5
	P3/HT	29	43×10^7	8	2129	$<0.2\text{-}200 \times 10^{-7}$	5.0
Lymph Nodes	729/HT	11	11×10^7	6	106	$<1.0\text{-}40 \times 10^{-7}$	0.8
	SP2/0	8	8×10^7	4	116	$<1.0\text{-}30 \times 10^{-7}$	1.5
	P3/HT	30	30×10^7	13	1852	$<1.0\text{-}200 \times 10^{-7}$	5.1
Tonsil	729/HT	2	2×10^7	1	18	$7.0\text{-}11 \times 10^{-7}$	0.9
	SP2/0	1	1×10^7	1	1	1.0×10^{-7}	0.1
	P3/HT	4	4×10^7	2	56	$8.0\text{-}30 \times 10^{-7}$	1.4
Spleen	729/HT	15	21×10^7	5	125	$0.3\text{-}30 \times 10^{-7}$	0.6
	ARH077	5	5×10^7	3	1	$1.0\text{-}1.0 \times 10^{-7}$	0.2
	GM607.11	4	4×10^7	2	2	$<1.0\text{-}2.0 \times 10^{-7}$	0.5
	SP2/0	5	5×10^7	3	104	$3.0\text{-}60 \times 10^{-7}$	2.1
	P3/HT	14	28×10^7	4	1389	$<0.2\text{-}100 \times 10^{-7}$	5.0

For each fusion, $1\text{-}3 \times 10^7$ lymphocytes were fused to $1\text{-}3 \times 10^7$ cells of the established human or mouse lymphoid tumor line. Cells were fused by the method of Gerhard[19] using 35% PEG 1000 + 7.5% DMSO and diluted into the appropriate HAT-selective medium.[11] Fused cells were plated into 96-well microtiter dishes at 10^5 cells/well without feeder layers. Growth medium for mouse-human hybrids was autoclavable MEM with 8% horse and 2% fetal calf serum; for human-human hybrids, the growth medium was RPMI 1640 plus 10% fetal calf serum.

Note: Due to plating density requirements, the maximum number of clones from any fusion was $20\text{-}40/10^6$ lymphocytes, or a fusion frequency of $200\text{-}400 \times 10^{-7}$.

can match or even exceed the fusion frequencies seen in mouse-mouse fusions (which range $1-2 \times 10^{-5}$). However, fusibility varies significantly not only among lymphocyte donors and tissue sources, but also for other reasons probably related to the condition of the cell line at the time of fusion. Despite rigorous attempts to treat the cell line uniformly, we found that 729/HT is not a completely reliable fusion partner for producing human hybridomas.

All three of the mouse myeloma lines, NS-1, SP2/0 and P3/HT, fused at least as well and usually better than 729/HT with the same lymphocyte preparations over many trials. In fact, most of the human lines fuse so poorly, relative to the mouse lines, that it was difficult to generate sufficient data to make other comparisons, such as yield of Ig-producing clones, Ig secretion rates, and stability. Thus we concentrated the rest of our study on the most fusible lines, the human lymphoblastoid line 729/HT, and the mouse myeloma P3/HT.

Yield of human Ig-secreting clones from fusions of P3/HT or 729/HT to human lymphocytes is presented in Table 3. Once again, lymphocyte variability is a major consideration: both specific donor and tissue source impact the final results of a fusion. We have calculated the yield of Ig-secreting clones over a large number of donors and tissue sources. The P3/HT parent yields higher numbers of Ig-producing clones than the human line 729/HT. In addition, there is the complication that 729/HT does produce its own IgM, although it secretes only low levels of the antibody (10^{-3} ng/ml). At this time, it is not possible to distinguish between those 729/HT hybridomas that are producing lymphocyte-derived or 729/HT-derived IgM. Therefore, the discrepancy in Ig-secreting clones produced by the mouse versus the human lymphoid tumor lines is probably greater than indicated in Table 3. We have also found (data not shown) that the range of Ig-secretion rates in 729/HT and P3/HT hybridomas is comparable, with a slight tendency of the P3/HT-human

Table 3
Immunoglobulin Production by Human-Human
and Mouse-Human Hybrids

Cell Line	pbls % IgM	pbls % IgG	Lymph Node % IgM	Lymph Node % IgG	Tonsil % IgM	Tonsil % IgG	Spleen % IgM	Spleen % IgG
729/HT	ND*	ND	23	13	28	0	20	6.7
P3/HT	28	2.3	68	23	25	7.6	55	31

*Not enough data available.

After two–three feedings, clone supernatants were assayed for the presence of human IgG or IgM by ELISA. Ig levels were determined by comparison to a polyclonal-IgG or IgM standard curve. Positive clones secreted greater than 0.1 μg/ml of human Ig.

Note: 729/HT produces low levels of IgM, but is surface Ig-positive. This screen does not distinguish between lymphocyte-derived and tumor line-derived IgM.

lymphocyte (mouse-human) hybridomas to produce more human Ig than 729/HT-human lymphocyte (human-human) hybridomas when made from the same lymphocyte pools.

With the mouse myeloma having a clear advantage in the first three critical areas of hybridoma production (fusibility, yield of Ig-production clones, and Ig secretion rate) it was necessary to measure the relative stability of the mouse-human versus human-human hybridomas. To generate stability data, we started with fusions of P3/HT and 729/HT in which clones grew in less than 33% of the microtiter wells used in the initial plating after fusion. This avoids the possibility that more than one hybrid initially grew in any given well, thereby limiting the chance the an Ig-producing clone would be lost by overgrowth of a non-Ig-producing clone. The stability analysis is complicated by residual lymphocyte antibody production, even several weeks after fusion and after several feedings. Figure 1 follows the relative stability of mouse-human and human-human hybrids over approximately a six-week period after identification of Ig-secreting clones. In general, clones that are positive at the freeze and/or subclone stage will remain positive or can be subcloned to produce a stable line. Thus, during the critical six-week period of stability analysis, a higher percentage of the P3/HT hybrids than the 729/HT hybrids remain stable for Ig production.

While the stability of the mouse-human hybrids was not especially surprising to us (from our previous work with the line), it was striking that the human-human hybrids were relatively unstable. This comparison of 729/HT and P3/HT led to two general conclusions. First, human-human hybrids are not necessarily more stable than interspecies hybrids. But it is quite possible that human lymphoid partners other than 729/HT might make more stable hybridomas. Second, mouse-human hybrids are not necessarily unstable. Stability appears to be a property of each individual parent line. Taking all of these considerations together — fusibility, Ig production, and stability — we concluded that the best way to produce specific human monoclonal antibodies by hybridoma technology was to use the P3/HT mouse myeloma line. An added inducement to the mouse-human system was that, in preliminary attempts, nine of 10 mouse-human hybrids, but none of 11 human-human hybrids tested could produce ascites in nude mice. Thus, it might be possible to produce large amounts of the human antibodies from such mouse-human hybridomas when grown as mouse ascites.

Sources of Immune Lymphocytes

There is substantial evidence that tumors are immunogenic in their hosts: for example, antitumor antibodies and/or immune complexes appear in the circulation, tumors are sometimes infiltrated with mononuclear

56

cells, and incidence of tumors is increased in immunodeficient patients. In fact, much early serotherapy was designed to bolster a patient's own immune system to reject the 'foreign' tumor tissue. We have therefore chosen to use lymphocytes from diagnosed tumor patients in order to produce human monoclonal antibodies to tumor-associated antigens, thereby assuming that these patients' immune systems have responded to their tumors.

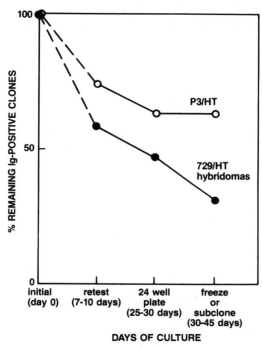

Figure 1 Stability of human Ig-secreting hybridomas made with P3/HT or 729/HT. Clones secreting greater than 0.1 ug/ml human IgG or IgM were identified by ELISA on culture supernatants three to five weeks after fusion, or when microtiter wells were approximately 1/3 confluent. Positive clones were transferred to second or 'retest' microtiter well and refed. Clones still postive at this stage were transferred to 24 well plates and allowed to regrow. When confluent, the supernatants of 24-well-plate wells were assayed again. Clones remaining positive were transferred to T-25 flasks, and were reassayed for Ig production prior to freezing or subcloning.

Notes: 1) Rapid initial loss of positive clones reflects presence of residual lymphocyte antibody in initial assay wells. Such antibody is diluted out by retest. Thus clones scoring positive at retest stage are assumed to be base line number of positives. 2) Clones represented in this diagram were derived from fusions with clone growth less than 30% of seeded wells. This removes the complication of multiple clones per well, and the possible loss of Ig activity due to overgrowth by non-Ig producing clones.

The most easily acquired human lymphocytes are those from peripheral blood. However, as Table 2 of our fusibility study demonstrates, peripheral blood is the least fusible source of lymphocytes due to the low numbers of activated cells in the circulation. Also as shown in Table 3, the yield of Ig-producing clones from pbls is relatively low. We therefore obtained lymphocytes from lymph nodes draining areas of solid tumors. When required as a part of a surgical procedure, lymph nodes were aseptically removed from the patient and placed in phosphate-buffered saline (PBS) at 4C. Lymphocytes were dissected out from the tissue as soon as possible, washed once in PBS, and were either fused immediately or frozen in liquid nitrogen for future work.

Production and Identification of Specific Antibodies to Tumor Cell Lines

Human monoclonal antibodies reactive with human breast tumor lines were derived by fusion of P3/HT to lymphocytes of lymph nodes draining breast tumors. The results of five such mouse-human fusions are shown in Table 4. Hybridoma supernatants were initially screened for production of human IgG or IgM by ELISA. Clones secreting more than 0.1 μg/ml human Ig were refed twice, then assayed for specific reactivity against a panel of three human breast tumor cell lines: T47D, MCF-7 and H925, and against the human foreskin fibroblast line 350Q as a negative control. The specific cell-surface ELISA was performed on whole cells glutaraldehyde-fixed in microtiter wells with a horseradish peroxidase (HRP) conjugated goat anti-human secondary reagent. Criteria for an initial screen-specific positive were set as an optical density greater then 0.5 (at 480 nm) on at least one of the breast cell lines and at least a five-fold

Table 4
Application of Mouse-Human Fusion Technology to Obtain Human Antibodies Recognizing Tumor Cells

Fusion	#P3/HT	# Lymph Node Lymphocytes	# Wells	# Clones	# IgG or IgM Positives	# Specific Positives*
YBA	10^7	10^7	200	112	50	1
YBB	2×10^7	2×10^7	400	286	146	2
YBC	2×10^7	2×10^7	400	149	55	2
YBD	4×10^7	3×10^7	700	242	40	1
YBE	4×10^7	3×10^7	800	119	33	0

*Specific positive were selected by the following criteria and screening protocols: 1) Human IgG or IgM production > 0.1 μg/ml as measured by ELISA. 2) Specific reactivity on breast tumor lines as measured by ELISA. Positives have > 0.5 O.D. on T47D or MCF-7 human breast tumor lines, and at least five-fold higher O.D. on one of these breast lines than on the 350Q foreskin fibroblast line.

stronger signal on a breast line than on the control 350Q line. Positive clones were transferred to larger wells of 24-well dishes and reassayed for specific activity. If still positive by the same criteria as for the initial specific screen, these clones were designated 'specific positives' and subjected to more extensive analysis. By these procedures we obtained six specific positive hybridomas out of 908 clones, or a specific positive frequency of 0.7%.

Four of the six hybridomas were selected for extensive analysis of reactivity patterns, stability, and potential for large-scale antibody production. All four of the antibodies are of the IgM class. To assess specificity, the four antibodies were assayed by cell surface ELISA against a panel of 16 cell lines, as shown in Table 5. Each antibody has a distinct pattern of reactivity. Three of the four antibodies show some crossreactivity with the small cell lung carcinoma line M103, and two of the four antibodies react with the T84 colon carcinoma line. YBD 047 and YBC 122 show greater specificity for the breast tumor lines and give only low signals when asayed on cell lines from other tissue sources.

Further analysis of tissue specificity is complicated by the human origin of the antibodies themselves. Human tumor and normal tissues con-

Table 5
Reactivity of Human Antibreast Monoclonal Antibodies Against Human Cell Lines

		ELISA OD (480 nm)			
		YBB190	YBC058	YBC122	YBD047
Origin	Cell Line	IgM	IgM	IgM	IgM
Mammary ca	T47D	>1.5	0.39	>1.5	0.95
Mammary ca	MCF-7	>1.5	0.23	0.63	0.45
Mammary ca	H925	0.06	0.03	0.18	0.03
Lung ca	H2540	0.70	0.17	0.25	0.14
Lung ad	A529	0.32	0.17	0.22	0.08
Lung, small cell	M103	>1.5	0.14	0.69	0.32
Lung, large cell	—	0.47	0.13	0.22	0.14
Colon ca	T84	1.45	0.23	0.19	0.18
Colon ca	SW480	0.27	0.08	0.12	0.08
Colon ca	320DM	0.18	0.14	0.55	0.15
Pancreatic	Panc-1	0.71	0.12	0.34	0.13
Neuroblastoma	SK-NSH	0.05	0.05	0.10	0.04
Melanoma	SK-Mel	0.07	0.07	0.35	0.12
Osteosarcoma	H998	0.12	0.31	0.21	0.14
Bladder ca	H907	0.29	0.10	0.37	0.06
Skin fibroblast	350Q	0.08	0.04	0.07	0.07

Culture supernatants were assayed by cell surface ELISA on glutaraldehyde-fixed whole cells. Antibody bound to cells was detected with HRP-conjugated goat antihuman Ig. Nonspecific IgM and IgG (human monoclonal) gave an O.D. reading <0.05.

tain large amounts of endogenous human immunoglobulin. Therefore, any analysis employing a labeled secondary antihuman Ig reagent will produce a nonspecific signal when the tracer is applied to human tissue. Second, the IgM antibodies themselves are very sticky, and will tend to bind nonspecifically to tissues, particularly to cytoplasms that have high concentrations of polyanions.

We are currently working to develop assay systems to test human antibodies on human tissue. Among potential solutions to this problem are: assay of human tumors grown in nude mice, direct coupling of human monoclonal antibodies to enzyme or radioisotopic labels (to avoid the endogenous Ig problem) and treatment of antibody and/or tissue with polycations, sugars, detergents, glycosidases, or other agents that might counteract the stickiness of the IgMs themselves. To date, we have obtained some favorable results with human breast tumors grown in nude mice. At least two of the human monoclonal antibodies, YBB190 and YBC058, react strongly with three different breast tumor models and do not react with a human melanoma tumor model when asayed by immunohistochemistry on cryostat blocks of the target tissue. This provides us with a preliminary indication that the specificity of these antibodies may carry over to a completely different assay system and target tissue, a result that is extremely encouraging.

While techniques are being developed to test specificity of these antibodies, we are continuing to monitor the stability of these hybridomas. All four of the human antibreast antibodies have been successfully subcloned (see Table 6). One, YBC 058.1 was subcloned a single time. The other three antibodies were subcloned twice in sequence to obtain good efficiency cloning. The parent and subclone populations of all four hybridomas have been stable in culture for over eight months. During those eight months, all four hybridomas have continued to make high levels of specifically reactive IgM antibody. Thus, we feel confident in our initial determination that hybridomas of P3/HT and human lymphocytes can be stable over a useful span of time. It should be noted that any hybridoma or cell line is expected to change over time in culture, and that, in order to maintain uniformity of a monoclonal antibody preparation, we routinely freeze large seed stocks of useful hybridomas and periodically return to the original stock to avoid drift of the cell population with continued culture.

The last issue, that of producing large amounts of human antibody, has been addressed by testing the ability of these mouse-human hybridomas to grow as nude mouse ascites. As shown in Table 6, all four of the human antibreast antibodies can grow as nude mouse ascites and produce human monoclonal antibodies. Antibody production is generally in the range of 1 mg/ml and titer of the antibodies on specific screen against the T47D breast cell line is in the range of 1/500–1/1000. Second passage titer

Table 6
Characterization of Human Monoclonal Antibodies
to Breast Tumor Cells

Hybridoma	Ig Class	Subcloned	Stability in Culture	Mouse Ascites	Comments
YBB 190	M	Twice	>8 mo	Positive to 1st passage	1st passage: IgM = 0.9 mg/ml; specific titer = 1:3000
YBC 058	M	Once	>8 mo	Positive to 2nd passage	1st passage: IgM = 1.0 mg/ml; specific titer = 1:1024
					2nd passage: IgM = 0.9 mg/ml; specific titer = 1:600
YBC 122	M	Twice	>8 mo	Positive to 1st passage	1st passage; IgM = 0.9 mg/ml; specific titer = 1:320
YBD 047	M	Twice	>8 mo	Positive to 1st passage	1st passage: IgM = 1.5 mg/ml; specific titer = 1:1600

Specific titer: Highest dilution that gives >25% of the maximum O.D. obtained with cell culture supernatant positive control when assayed by cell surface ELISA on the T47D breast cell line.

generally declines. We are therefore studying various ways of pretreating the hybridoma cells and/or the host mice to maintain antibody production in subsequent passages. However, at this time in vivo human antibody production in ascites can yield milligram quantities of antibody. We are therefore within reach of our goal to produce large amounts of specifically reactive human monoclonal antibodies, and we can begin to test the usefulness of these antibodies in a clinical setting. It will be particularly important to learn if these antibodies will generate an immune response by the patient (particularly anti-idiotype), and whether this response neutralizes the efficacy of a human antibody-based pharmaceutical. If human antibodies can eliminate the problems encountered in clinical trials of mouse monoclonal antibodies, then they will surely earn an important place in immunotherapy in the future.

ACKNOWLEDGMENTS

The authors would like to thank Joli Diveley, Joanie Hayden, Diane Joergensen, Julia Leung, Dan Mackensen, Lana Rittmann and Mike Unger and many others at Hybritech for their contributions to this research, and Karyl LaPinska for typing this manuscript.

REFERENCES

1. Paul WE, Sredni B, Schwartz RH: Long-term growth and cloning of non-transformed lymphocytes. *Nature* 1981;294:697–699.
2. Leanderson T, Lundgren E, Ruuth E, et al: B-cell growth factor: Distinction from T-cell growth factor and B-cell maturation factor. *Proc Natl Acad Sci* 1982;79:7455–7459.
3. Butler JL, Lane HC, Fauci AS: Delineation of optimal conditions for producing mouse-human heterohybridomas from human peripheral blood B cells of immunized subjects. *J Immunol* 1983;130:165–168.
4. Butler JL, Muraguchi A, Lane HC, et al: Development of a human T-T cell hybridoma secreting B cell growth factor. *J Exp Med* 1983;157:60–68.
5. Kehrl JH, Fauci AS: Identification, purification, and characterization of antigen-activated and antigen-specific human B lymphocytes. *J Exp Med* 1983;157:1692–1697.
6. Rosen A, Persson K, Klein G: Human monoclonal antibodies to a genus-specific chlamydial antigen, produced by EBV-transformed B cells. *J Immunol* 1983;130:2899–2902.
7. Winger L, Winger C, Shastry P, et al: Efficient generation in vitro, from human peripheral blood cells, of monoclonal Epstein-Barr virus transformants producing specific antibody to a variety of antigens without prior deliberate immunization. *Proc Natl Acad Sci* 1983;80:4484–4488.
8. Monjour L, Desgranges C, Alfred C, et al: Production of human monoclonal antibodies against asexual erythrocytic stages of *Plasmodium falciparum*. *Lancet* 1983;1337–1338.
9. Watson DB, Burns GF, Mackay IR: In vitro growth of B lymphocytes infiltrating human melanoma tissue by transformation with EBV: Evidence for secretion of anti-melanoma antibodies by some transformed cells. *J Immunol* 1983;130:2442–2447.
10. Kohler G, Milstein C: Continuous cultures of fused cells secreting antibody of pre-defined specificity. *Nature* 1975;256:495–497.
11. Littlefield JW: Selection of hybrids from matings of fibroblasts in vitro and their presumed recombinants. *Science* 1964;145:709–710.
12. Olsson L, Kaplan HS: Human-human hybridomas producing monoclonal antibodies of predefined antigenic specificity. *Proc Natl Acad Sci* 1980;77:5429–5434.
13. Cote RJ, Morrissey DM, Houghton AN, et al: Generation of human monoclonal antibodies reactive with cellular antigens. *Proc Natl Acad Sci* 1983;80:2026–2030.
14. Pickering JW, Gelder FB: A human myeloma cell line that does not express immunoglobulin but yields a high frequency of antibody-secreting hybridomas. *J Immunol* 1982;129:406–412.
15. Abrams PG, Knost JA, Clarke G, et al: Determination of the optimal human cell lines for development of human hybridomas. *J Immunol* 1983;131:1201–1204.
16. Nowinski R, Berglund C, Lane J, et al: Human monoclonal antibody against Forssman antigen. *Science* 1980;210:537–538.
17. Schlom J, Wunderlich D, Teramoto YA: Generation of human monoclonal antibodies reactive with human mammary carcinoma cells. *Proc Natl Acad Sci* 1980;77:6841–6845.
18. Lever JR, Nuki G, Seegmiller JE: *Proc Natl Acad Sci* 1979;71:2679–2683.
19. Gerhard W, in Kennett R, McKearn TJ, Bechtol KG (eds): *Monoclonal Antibodies*. New York, Plenum Press, 1980, p 370.

6 Production, Purification and Biochemical Characterization of Monoclonal Antibodies Reacting with Human Breast Carcinoma Cells

R. Mandeville, J. Lecomte, F. M. Sombo J. Chausseau, L. Giroux

The purpose of this study was the production of monoclonal antibodies (MCAs) that react with a high degree of specificity to human breast cancer cells for a potential use in tumor diagnosis and/or therapy. MCAs were produced by fusing Ns-1 myeloma cells to spleen cells from BALB/c mice hyperimmunized with the well-characterized human breast carcinoma cell line BT-20. Hybridoma were selected on the basis of their preferential binding in an ELISA assay to human mammary tumor cells. Stable MCA-producing lines were isolated by cloning. Determination of immunoglobulin (Ig) class and subclass showed that five of these hybridoma cultures synthesized IgG1 and only one IgG2 isotype. Levels of Ig synthesis ranged from 81.15 to 136.65 μg/ml in the supernatant fluids. Ammonium sulphate precipitation and ion-exchange chromatography allowed the isolation of partially purified material that was further used as a possible tool to distinguish breast carcinoma cells from normal cells of the same histogenesis. For these studies, three different techniques were used: ELISA, dot-immunobinding, and indirect immunofluorescence. Immunochemical analysis showed that these MCAs recognize protein determinants on the cell surface membrane since their reactivity was unaffected by treatment with neuraminidase or by lipid extraction, while it was completely destroyed by proteinase K and trypsin treatments. Moreover, in the case of four of these MCAs the identification of a glycoprotein moiety could be established. Preliminary studies on tumor biopsies showed that these MCAs react with a high degree of specificity to human mammary carcinoma cells.

The advent of the hybridoma technology[1] for the production of large amounts of high titered monoclonal antibodies (MCAs) with a unique specificity for the antigen has greatly improved the possibility of probing the cell-surface antigenic complex of tumor cells and spurred efforts to generate tumor-specific antibodies. Investigators have used a variety of approaches for producing McAs that recognize various antigenic structures on malignant and/or normal breast tissues.[2-18] In this communication, we describe the use of hybridoma technology to generate a panel of hybridoma-secreting monoclonal antibodies that react with a high degree of specificity to human breast cancer cells. The potential of these MCAs to probe surface protein differences between normal and malignant breast cancer cells will also be described. BT-20 breast carcinoma cell line was used as our source of antigens because it was derived from a poorly differentiated tumor[19] and has been well characterized and extensively studied.[20-26] More importantly for our studies, these cells were very tumorigenic when implanted in the nude athymic mice, producing nodules with the same morphologic characteristics as the original tumor.[21] These cells seem to have kept the properties of breast carcinoma.

MATERIAL AND METHODS

Cultured Cell Lines

A nonimmunoglobulin-producing murine myeloma cell line NS-1 (P3.NS/2.Ag4.1) was obtained from the Cell Distribution Center at the Salk Institute, San Diego, CA.[27] BT-20 and HBL-100 cell lines were both obtained from Dr. A.E. Bogden, Mason Research Institute, Rockville, MD.

Tests for mycoplasma contamination using direct agar culture were performed by Dr. C. Hours (Quality Control Lab., Institut Armand-Frappier) and only negative lines were used in this study. All cell lines were maintained in RPMI-1640 (Flow Lab) supplemented with 10% fetal calf serum (GIBCO), 0.01 M Hepes buffer pH 7.4, 100 IU/ml penicillin, 100 μg/ml streptomycin, and 100 μg/ml gentamycin sulfate (Microbiological Associates).

Hyperimmunization

Female BALB/c mice (6–8 weeks old) were immunized with three weekly sc injections of 1–2 $\times$ 10^7 BT-20 cells, with the initial immunization in complete Freunds̄ adjuvant. For all the immunizations, BT-20 cells were cultured in serum-free medium for 24 hours before harvesting, and were detached from the culture vessel by means of a rubber policeman. Rise in serum antibody titers in immunized mice was monitored weekly and animals showing high response to BT-20 were selected. The booster dose was given ip only when the antibody titer dropped back to base-line levels, ie, 27 days after the third immunization.

Cell Fusion and Cloning

Spleen cells from hyperimmunized animals were mixed with NS-1 cells at a ratio of 5:1, and the cell mixture (after pelleting and centrifugation) was resuspended in 0.1 ml of 50% (w/v) polyethylene glycol 1000 (BDH Chemicals, Ltd., England) in serum-free RPNI-1640. Visible hybridomas appeared four to five days after fusion. After six days of culture they were fed hypoxanthine-aminopterin-thymidine (HAT) medium without fetal calf serum, and after nine days, RPMI-1640 only. Cultures selected for their preferential binding to BT-20 were cloned by limiting dilution in the presence of 3T3 fibroblasts as feeder layer. After further characterization, the selected hybridomas were expanded in complete media and injected ip into pristane-primed BALB/c mice for the production of ascitic fluid.

Biochemical Analysis and Purification

The heavy and light chain composition of MCAs was determined using Ouchterlony gels, first against affinity-purified goat-antiserum specific for each of murine subclasses (IgG1, IgG2a, IgG2b, IgG3, IgM and IgA), and then to monospecific goat-antimouse immunoglobulin isotypes (Cappel Lab., Cochranville, PA). Quantitation of MCAs was performed by a standard radioimmunoassay using goat antimouse IgG (Miles Laboratories). Purification of ascitic fluids was performed by precipitation with 55% saturated $(NH_4)^2SO_4$ pH 7.3 followed by solubilization and extensive dialysis against Tris-HCl 0.01M, pH 8.0 in the cold (Figure 1). Further purification was obtained by chromatography on QAE-Sephadex column (Pharmacia, Uppsala, Sweden) equilibrated in Tris-HCl 0.01 M pH 8.0, using a gradient of 0–0.5 M sodium chloride.

ELISA Assay

Analysis and quantitation of MCAs were performed using an enzyme-linked immunosorbent assay (ELISA). Glutaraldehyde fixed BT-20 or HBL-100 cells were used as antigens. They were overlayed with 50 μl of hybridoma supernatant and allowed to incubate for 30 minutes at 37C in a humidified atmosphere. After three washes, 50 μl of horseradish peroxidase-labeled goat antimouse IgG (New England Nuclear) diluted 1:500 in PBS-Tween, was added to each well and incubated for 45 minutes at 37C. The amount of peroxidase bound to fixed cells was determined by using 0.2% O-phenylenediamine and hydrogen peroxide. Absorbance at 492 nm was measured with a Titertek multiskan photometer (Flow Lab). All data were expressed as a mean reading of three test samples minus the reading of control culture.

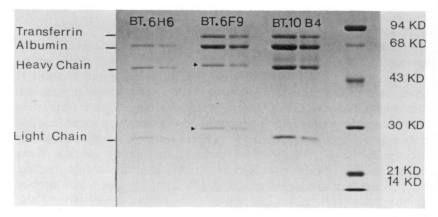

Figure 1 SDS-PAGE profile of three monoclonal antibodies partially purified by precipitation with 55% saturated ammonium sulfate. It should be noted that BT.6 F9 (IgG2a) showed consistently heavier Ig chains (arrowhead) than IgG1 isotypes. Bio-Rads molecular weight standards consist of a series of natural proteins with molecular weight ranging from 14 KD (lysozyme) to 94 KD (phosphorylase B).

Dot-Immunobinding Detection of Antigens on Polyvinyl Chloride Membranes

Confluent monolayers were briefly washed in deionized water and collected by means of a rubber policeman, adjusted to a concentration of about 5×10^4 cells/ml and subjected to two cycles of freeze thawing to disrupt the cells. Two to three microliters of this suspension were dotted onto polyvinyl chloride filters. The antigen-dotted filter could be stored dry for several weeks without any loss of activity. Unoccupied binding sites were quenched by incubation in 1% polyvinyl-pyrolidone (Sigma, MW 40000) for one hour at 37C. The filters were then overlaid with 0.2 ml of hybridoma culture fluid for two hours at room temperature, washed five times for a period of 30 minutes each in PBS-Tween and quenched again with 1% polyvinyl-pyrolidone. Filters were then incubated for two hours in 0.2 ml of horseradish peroxidase-labeled goat antimouse IgG (New England Nuclear) diluted 1/1000 and revealed by 0.2% O-phenylene-dideamine, and hydrogen peroxide at room temperature and in a dark chamber. Positive reactions were revealed by a dark spot on a white background and reactivity graded from negative to 3+.

Indirect Immunofluorescence

Cell lines in logarithmic growth phase were washed twice in medium, air dried, and fixed in cold acetone for five minutes. Tumor tissues obtained from patients undergoing surgery were frozen in liquid nitrogen and 6- to 8-μm sections were prepared from the frozen samples in a cryostat. Representative sections of each tumor were stained with H & E and the presence of tumor cells was confirmed. Cells and/or tissue sections were incubated for 20 minutes at room temperature with hybridoma supernatant diluted 1/25 in PBS, then for 30 minutes in fluorescein-labeled goat anti-mouse IgG (Cappel Lab., Cochanville, PA) diluted 1/50 in PBS. These concentrations were used because they gave clear positive reactivity and total absence of any unwanted background. After two washes in PBS for 10 minutes, the slides were mounted with 50% glycerol in PBS, examined, and photographed with a Zeiss fluorescent microscope (Carl Zeiss, NY).

Treatment of Antigens by Chemicals and Enzymes

All treatments were performed on the antigens (BT-20 cell suspensions) immobilized on polyvinyl chloride filters, right after the first quenching with polyvinyl-pyrolidone. Aliquots containing 2–3 μl of 10^4 cells/ml were treated for 60 minutes at 37C with either proteinase K (2 mg/ml), trypsin (0.25%) or neuraminidase (0.1 Unit/ml). Periodate oxidation was carried out at room temperature for 60 minutes with 50 mM sodium metaperiodate in PBS adjusted to pH 6.0. Total lipid extraction was performed by treatment with a mixture of chloroform and methanol (1:2 by volume) using standard procedures.[28]

RESULTS AND DISCUSSION

Spleen cells from mice hyperimmunized with BT-20 cells were fused with the murine myeloma cell line NS/1. Five days after fusion, 100% of the seeded culture wells showed positive growth. Supernatant from these cultures were repeatedly screened by the ELISA technique to ensure reactivity to BT-20. In the initial assays, 40% of the culture wells secreted antibodies binding to the immunizing cell line, BT-20. As a first screening for specificity, culture fluids were comparatively tested against HBL-100 cell line, a normal human epithelial cell derived from milk sample. Only 18% of the hybrids were selected on the basis of their preferential binding to BT-20 cells but not to their normal counterpart, ie, HBL-100. Hybridomas were cloned and subcloned. Six positive clones were further expanded and reinjected intraperitoneally to pristane-primed BALB/c mice for the production of ascitic fluid. Isotype analysis revealed that five antibodies were of the IgG1 class, and that antibody BT.6F9 represents IgG2 immunoglobulin (Table 1). All MCAs also produced k light chain. Quantification of the immunoglobulin showed that these MCAs produced exceptionally high titers of IgG in the supernatant fluid ranging from 19.61

to 136.65 µg/ml (Table 1). Isolation of partially purified material was achieved by ammonium sulphate precipitation and analyzed by SDS-polyacrylamide gel electrophoresis (Figure 1). It was observed that IgG2a MCAs possess substantially heavier Ig chains (heavy and light chains) than IgG1 isotypes. The reactivity of the six purified MCAs was further tested using three different techniques: the ELISA assay, the Dot-immunoblotting assay, and fluorescence. We could show strong similarities in the pattern of reaction of all MCAs ie, strong reactivity to BT-20 cells, and no or low reactivity to HBL-100 (Table 2).

Immunochemical Analysis of the Determinant Recognized by Each Monoclonal Antibody

In these experiments, BT-20 cells were exposed to different chemicals or enzymes and then tested for residual antigenic activity with each MCA using the dot-immunoblotting assay. The effects of the removal of lipids as well as the reactions of these preparations with periodate, proteinase K, trypsin, and neuraminidase are reported in Figure 2. MCA-defined antigen were stable after treatment with neuraminidase, whereas it was com-

Table 1
Characteristics of Cloned Hybridoma Produced Monoclonal Antibodies

MCA	Ig Class	Ig (µg/ml)
BT.6 F9	IgG2a, k	81.15
BT.6 H6	IgG1, k	88.00
BT.6 D7	IgG1, k	19.61
BT.10 B4	IgG1, k	126.00
BT.10 H1	IgG1, k	108.90
BT.10 G2	IgG1, k	135.65

Table 2
Comparative Reactivity of Selected Monoclonal Antibodies to BT-20 and HBL-100 Using Three Different Techniques

	Reactivity					
	ELISA*		Dot-Immunobinding		Fluorescence	
MCA	BT-20	HBL-100	BT-20	HBL-100	BT-20	HBL-100
BT.6 F9	2+	1+	3+	1+	3+	−
BT.6 H6	1+	−	1+	−	1+	−
BT.6 D7	1+	−	2+	−	2+	−
BT.10 B4	2+	−	3+	−	3+	−
BT.10 H1	3+	1+	3+	−	2+	−
BT.10 G2	2+	1+	3+	−	3+	−

*Optical density (492 nm) ≥ 0.8 = 3+, 0.6 − 0.4 = 2+, 0.4 − 0.2 = 1+, ≤ 0.2 = −ve.

pletely abolished by treatment with proteinase K and trypsin. Moreover, removal of lipids from cell suspensions had no apparent effect. These results suggested a protein nature of the antigens recognized by all six MCAs. Moreover, four of these antibodies seem to identify a glycoprotein moiety since they showed strong sensitivity to periodate treatment (Figure 2).

Reactivity of Monoclonal Antibodies with Normal and Cancerous Epithelial Cells

Immunofluorescence data using a pool of the six MCAs selected, or each MCA separately, indicated that they identify a cell membrane structure present on mammary cancerous epithelial cells and not on their normal counterpart, HBL-100 (Figure 3). In addition, these MCAs were tested against a panel of carcinomas (breast, lung, endometrial, and endocervical) and normal breast tissue. These studies showed that they react with 100% of the primary breast carcinoma tested and/or their metastatic invasions of the lymph nodes. On the other hand, with the exception of the low reactivity noticed with one endometrial carcinoma, all other carcinomas tested bound background level of fluorescence. It was also noted that MCAs do not react with normal cells or connective tissue surrounding the malignant cells within the same biopsy and normal breast tissues.

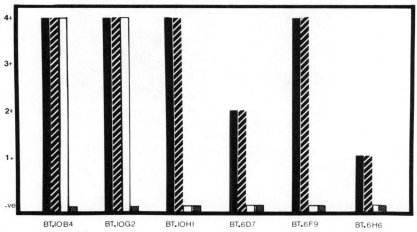

Figure 2 Characterization of antigens recognized by each MCA. Reactivity of the different monoclonal antibodies with BT-20 cells after treatment with enzymes or chemicals was compared to corresponding reactivity without pretreatment (solid column) using the Dot-immunobinding assay. No effect was seen when cells were pretreated with neuraminidase or methanol: chloroform (2:1) (striped column) while proteinase K and trypsin (open column) completely abolished this reactivity. With periodate treatment (dotted column) only BT.10 B4 and BT.10 H1 retain their reactivity.

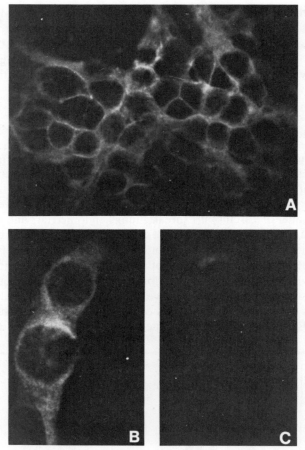

Figure 3 Human breast carcinoma cells showing strong reactivity with a pool of the six MCAs selected. Note the positive reaction on the cytoplasmic membrane of BT-20 cells (A and B) and the lack of staining in normal epithelial cells derived from human milk sample (C) × 500 for A and × 1000 for B and C.

CONCLUSION

We have produced a panel of MCAs that show a strong specificity to breast carcinoma cells binding mainly to cell-surface structures, identified biochemically to be of a protein or a glycoprotein moiety. Preliminary data on their clincial use showed an almost exclusive binding to breast cancer cells. Further studies are in progress to identify the molecular structure of the epitope recognized as well as the biological activities of each of the MCAs selected.

REFERENCES

1. Kohler G, Milstein C: *Nature* 1975;256:495–497.
2. Ceriani RL, Thompson K, et al: *Proc Natl Acad Sci* 1977;74:582–586.
3. Taylor-Papadimitriou J, Peterson JA, Arklie J, et al: *Int J Cancer* 1981;28: 17–21.
4. Sasaki M, Peterson JA, Ceriani RL: *Hybridoma* 1983;2:120.
5. Colcher D, Hand PH, Nuti M, et al: *Proc Natl Acad Sci* 1981;78:3199–3203.
6. Soule HR, Linder E, Edgington TS: *Proc Natl Acad Sci* 1983;80:1332–1336.
7. Crawford LV, Pim DC, et al: *J Proc Natl Acad Sci* 1981;78:41–45.
8. Kufe DW, Nadler L, et al: *Cancer Res* 1983;43:851–857.
9. Schlom J, Wunderlich D, Teramoto YA: *Proc Natl Acad Sci* 1980;77: 6841–6845.
10. Menard S, Tagliabue E, Canevari S, et al: *Cancer Res* 1983;43:1295–1300.
11. Canevari S, Fossati G, Balsari A: *Cancer Res* 1983;43:1301–1305.
12. Papsidero LD, Nemoto T, Valenzuela LA, et al: *Hybridoma* 1982;1:275–284.
13. Papsidero LD, Croghan GA, et al: *Cancer Res* 1983;43:1741–1747.
14. Yuan D, Hendler FJ, Vitetta ES: *J Natl Cancer Inst* 1982;68:719–728.
15. Mariani-Costantini R, Menard S, Clemente C, et al: *J Clin Path* 1982;35:1037.
16. Mariani-Costantini R, Della Torre G, Deotti TG, et al (eds): *Membrane in Tumor Growth*. New York, Elsevier Biochemical Press, 1982, pp 583–589.
17. Foster CS, Edwards PAW, Dinsdale EA, et al: *Virchows Arch [Pathol Anat]* 1982;394:279–293.
18. Foster CS, Dinsdale EA, Edwards PAW, et al: *Virchows Arch [Pathol Anat]* 1982;394:295–305.
19. Lasfargues EY, Ozzello L: *J Natl Cancer Inst* 1958;21:1131–1147.
20. Lasfargues EY, Coutinho WG, Moore DH: *Cancer Res* 1972;32:2365–2368.
21. Ozello L, Sordat B, et al: *J Natl Cancer Inst* 1974;52:1669–1672.
22. Ozello L, Lasfargues EY, Murray MR: *Cancer Res* 1960;20:600–605.
23. Buehring GC, Hackett AJ: *J Natl Cancer Inst* 1974;53:621–629.
24. Sinkovics JG, Reeves WJ, Cabiness JR: *J Natl Cancer Inst* 1972;48:1145–1149.
25. Jeejee Bhoy HF: *Br J Cancer* 1977;35:161–169.
26. Hurlimann J, Dayal R: *J Natl Cancer Inst* 1978;61:677–686.
27. Kearney JF, Radbruch A, Liesegang B, et al: *J Immunol* 1979;123:1548–1550.
28. Tettamanti G, Bonali F, Marchesini S, et al: *Biochem Biophys Acta* 1980; 296:160–170.

7 Monoclonal Antibodies to Human Small-Cell Lung Cancer

L. S. Rittmann, R. E. Sobol,
R. W. Astarita, J. Martinis

Mouse monoclonal antibodies reactive with human small-cell lung cancer (SCLC) were produced by two protocols. In the first protocol, spleen cells from mice immunized with the small-cell lung line, M103, were fused with the murine myeloma line, SP2/0. Using an enzyme-linked immunoassay (ELISA), 85 hybridomas were selected from four fusions that demonstrated a fivefold or greater activity on the small-cell lung line than on a bladder carcinoma line. Twenty-four of these were screened against a panel of human tumor cell lines. Four monoclonal antibodies out of 24 examined reacted exclusively with the small-cell lung lines. Other clones showed cross-reactivities most frequently with colon and breast carcinoma or neuroblastoma cell lines. In the second protocol, monoclonal antibodies to the small-cell tumor marker bombesin were produced by fusing spleen cells from bombesin-immunized mice with the murine myeloma line P3.653. These hybridomas were screened for reactivity with bombesin by ELISA and radioimmunoassay (RIA). Specific positives were screened on panels of human tumor lines and demonstrated reactivity with the small-cell lines. Antibodies derived from both protocols were examined by immunoperoxidase staining on frozen sections of small-cell lung carcinomas. LSA 285, a small-cell antibody, and BBA 078, a bombesin antibody, both stained frozen sections of small cell lung tumors.

Monoclonal antibodies to small-cell lung cancer may offer a valuable supplement to the current treatment of the disease. Small-cell lung cancer is a highly metastatic neoplasm, which is directly related to its extreme lethality. Antibodies capable of targeting metastatic lesions and delivering drug, toxin or radiation may be of considerable value in the treatment of this disease, which is generally not amenable to surgical resection. We have produced monoclonal antibodies cell-surface antigens present on human small-cell lung carcinomas as well as to the small-cell tumor marker, bombesin. Bombesin is a neuropeptide present in high concentrations in small-cell tumor lung lines and small-cell tumors.[1,2] The reactivities of these antibodies against cell lines as well as frozen sections of small-cell tumor were examined.

MATERIALS AND METHODS

Immunizations

Mice were immunized with two intraperitoneal injections of 5×10^6 M103 small-cell lung cancer cells, or with two intraperitoneal injections of 100 μg Lys[3]-bombesin (Peninsula Laboratories) conjugated to carrier protein. Mice were boosted four days prior to fusion with the immunizing antigen. Spleen cells were fused with SP2/0 and P3.653 mouse myeloma cells according to the procedure of Gerhard et al.[3]

ELISA and RIA Screens

Tumor cell lines, which grow as monolayers, were placed in microtiter plates and allowed to grow overnight. The following day they were fixed with 0.0125% glutaraldehyde. Nonadherent cell lines were plated out in poly L-lysine coated microwell plates, centrifuged for five minutes at 150 g, and fixed with 0.2% glutaraldehyde in phosphate-buffered saline at 4C according to the method of Cobbold and Waldman.[4]

Antibombesin hybridomas were screened by both ELISA and RIA. For the ELISA assay, bombesin was dried onto microtiter plates at 5 ng/well. Forty microliters of hybridoma supernatant was added and allowed to incubate for one hour at 37C. Plates were washed and incubated with peroxidase-conjugated goat antimouse immunoglobulin. Positive clones were identified by subsequent addition of 100 μl of 1 mg/ml OPD, 0.1% hydrogen peroxide, citrate-phosphate buffer pH 5.0. [TyR[4]]-bombesin (Peninsula Laboratories, Belmont, CA) was iodinated utilizing chloramine T and was used as the tracer for the RIA.

Immunoperoxidase Staining of Tissue

Fresh frozen small-cell autopsy tissue was utilized for immunohistochemistry. Sections were reacted with primary antibody for two hours, washed extensively with phosphate-buffered saline, and then incubated with peroxidase-conjugated goat antimouse immunoglobulin. Color development followed the addition of 0.6 mg/ml diaminobenzidine, phosphate-buffered saline in the presence of dilute hydrogen peroxide.

RESULTS AND DISCUSSION

A summary of the M103 small-cell lung fusions is shown in Table 1. Clones were designated as positive when they displayed a fivefold or greater reactivity with the NCI H69 small-cell line than with the H907 bladder carcinoma cell line. The positive clones were screened again utiliz-

Table 1
Summary of Small-Cell Lung Carcinoma and Bombesin Fusions

| Fusion Code | Clone Production | | Retest Positives | |
	Number of Clones	Number of Clones / Total Wells Plated	Number of Retest Positives	Retest Positives / Total Clones
LSA	336	23%	25	7%
LSB	39	5%	13	33%
LSC	308	16%	23	8%
LSD	681	64%	142	21%
BBA	98	12%	6	6%
BBC	483	32%	23	5%

Table 2
Screening Monoclonal Antibodies on a Panel of Fixed Human Cells
OD 490/30 Minutes in Solid-Phase Enzyme-Linked Binding Away

| Cell Lines | | SCLC Monoclonal Antibodies | | | |
		LSA 285	LSA 289	LSA 108	LSA 280
Small cell	M103	.33	.39	.14	.17
Small cell	NCI H69	.51	1.39	.20	.29
Lung adenocarcinoma	CH27LCI	.03	.07	.05	.01
Lung squamous	H928	.02	.02	.04	.02
Lung large	H2540	.04	.02	.10	.03
Mammary carcinoma	T47D	.04	.06	.08	.05
Mammary carcinoma	MCF7	.02	.01	.03	.04
Bladder carcinoma	H907	.01	.01	.07	.02
Melanoma	SkMel	.07	.04	.00	.06
Neuroblastoma	TE671	.00	.01	.00	.06
Neuroblastoma	SKNSH	.06	.02	.06	.02
Colon carcinoma	Colo320	.05	ND	ND	ND
Fibroblast	350Q	.01	.00	.01	.03

ND = not determined.

ing identical assay procedures. Retest positive clones ranged from 7% of total clones in fusion LSA to 33% in fusion LSB. Clone production and percent retest positives for two bombesin fusions is also shown in Table 1. Antibombesin retest positives included clones that displayed differential reactivity in the ELISA and RIA screens.

The reactivities of four small-cell positive monoclonal antibodies against a panel of human tumor cell lines are shown in Table 2. The antibodies demonstrate relative specificity for the small-cell lung tumor lines in this assay. Table 3 shows four other antibodies that showed limited reactivities to other human tumor cell lines. LSA 074 crossreacted with

Table 3
Screening Monoclonal Antibodies on a Panel of Fixed Human Cells
OD 490/30 Minutes in Solid-Phase Enzyme-Linked Binding Assay

Cell Lines		SCLC Monoclonal Antibodies			
		LSA 074	LSA 062	LSA 283	LSA 286
Small cell	M103	>1.5	.30	>1.5	>1.5
Small cell	NCI H69	1.32	.20	>1.5	1.4
Lung adenocarcinoma	CH27LCI	.00	.05	.03	.18
Lung squamous	H928	.00	.05	.06	ND
Mammary carcinoma	T47D	.02	.05	.10	.76
Mammary carcinoma	MCF7	.16	.02	.37	1.04
Bladder carcinoma	H907	.05	.01	.05	.11
Melanoma	SkMel	.00	.07	.06	.01
Neuroblastoma	TE671	.00	.05	.06	.00
Neuroblastoma	SKNSH	.75	.09	.88	.00
Colon carcinoma	T84	1.20	.07	ND	.10
Fibroblast	350Q	.00	.00	.04	.01
Lung large	H2540	.02	.22	.07	.03

ND = not determined.

a neuroblastoma cell line and a colon carcinoma cell line. LSA 062 crossreacted with the large-cell lung line. This is interesting in view of recent observations by Gazdar et al,[5] who described conversions of small-cell-derived lung lines to large-cell-type morphology in cell culture. LSA 283 reacted very strongly with both small-cell lines, but much more weakly with the mammary carcinoma line, MCF7, and the neuroblastoma line, SKNSH. LSA 286 reacted with both mammary carcinoma cell lines examined. The high affinity bombesin monoclonal antibody, BBA 078, was tested in a similar multicell screen. It reacted with both small-cell lung lines (Table 4). It also reacted weakly with the large-cell lung line, the neuroblastoma line, and the colon carcinoma line.

The small-cell associated antibodies that demonstrated specificity in the multicell assay were examined on frozen sections of small-cell tumors obtained at autopsy. LSA 285, 286 and 283 all stained frozen sections of small-cell tumors. BBA 078 was screened on a panel of normal and neoplastic tissue (Table 5), BBA 078 intensely stained all small-cell tumors examined. It did not react with normal liver, kidney or breast tissue. BBA 078 reacted with the majority of other non-small-cell lung carcinomas examined, including adrenocarcinoma, epidermoid carcinoma and large cell carcinoma. It also reacted with normal colon and the bronchial epithelium of one normal lung.

SUMMARY

We have identified monoclonal antibodies that demonstrated specificity to small-cell lung cancer in cell line ELISA assays. These antibodies

Table 4
Reactivity of Antibombesin Monoclonal (BBA 078) Against Tumor Cell Lines OD 490/30 Minutes in Solid-Phase Enzyme-Linked Binding Assay

Tumor Line		ELISA OD 490 nm
Small cell	M103	.30
Small cell	NCIH69	.24
Squamous carcinoma lung	CALU-1	.05
Adenocarcinoma lung	CH27LCI	.02
Large cell lung	H2540	.11
Bladder carcinoma	H907	.03
Mammary carcinoma	T47D	.05
Mammary carcinoma	BT-20	.04
Pancreatic carcinoma	PANC-1	.03
Prostatic carcinoma	PC3	.02
Prostatic carcinoma	DU145	.07
Melanoma	SKMEL	.05
Melanoma	BROWN	.02
Neuroblastoma	SKNSH	.18
Colon carcinoma	COLO 320 DM	.12
Fibroblast	350Q	.02
Fibroblast	WIL	.04

Table 5
Immunoperoxidase Staining of Antibombesin Monoclonal Antibody (BBA 078) on Normal and Tumor Tissue

Small cell lung tumors	3/3
Adenocarcinoma of lung	4/5
Epidermoid carcinoma of lung	5/6
Large cell lung carcinoma	2/3
Normal lung	1/2
Normal kidney	0/1
Normal breast	0/1
Normal liver	0/1
Normal colon	1/1

also react with frozen sections of small-cell tumor tissue. Although these antibodies did not exhibit complete specificity for the target tumor in frozen section assays, they may still prove valuable for the in vivo imaging of tumors and the immunotherapy of the disease. In addition, a panel of these antibodies could aid the evaluation of bone marrow biopsies in diagnosing the disease, as well as the phenotyping of various tumors by immunohistology. Finally, bombesin-like peptides have been shown to exist in the serum of patients with extensive disease. The generation of high affinity monoclonal antibodies should improve the ability to detect this antigen and make serum diagnosis of early stage disease and serum monitoring feasible.

ACKNOWLEDGMENTS

We thank John Alaimo, William Soo Hoo, Rene Lampa, Jim Myers and Chris Hofeditz for technical assistance.

REFERENCES

1. Moody TW, Pert CB, Gazdar AF, et al: High Levels of Intracellular bombesin characterize human small-cell lung carcinoma. *Science* 1981;214:1246.
2. Wood SM, Wood JR, Ghatei MA, et al: Bombesin, somatostatin and neurotension-like immunoreactivity in bronchial carcinoma. *J Clin Endocrinol Metab* 1981;53:1310.
3. Gerhard W, in Kennett R, McKearn TJ, Bechtol KG (eds): *Monoclonal Antibodies*. New York, Plenum Press, 1980, p 370.
4. Cobbold SP, Waldmann H: A rapid solid-phase enzyme-linked binding assay for screening monoclonal antibodies to cell surface antigens. *J Immunol Methods* 1981;44:125.
5. Gazdar AF, Carney DN, Guccion JG, et al: Small cell carcinoma of lung: Cellular origin and relationship to other pulmonary tumors, in Greco FA, Oldham RK, Bunn PA, (eds): *Small Cell Carcinoma of the Lung*. New York, Grune and Stratton, 1981; p 145.

8 Prophylactic Treatment of Kidney Transplant Recipients with a Monoclonal Anti-T Cell Antibody (OKT3-PAN)

P. Vigeral, M. Chkoff, L. Chatenoud,
D. Droz, J. Schindler, G. Goldstein,
M. Lacombe, C. Choquenet, J. F. Bach,
H. Kreis

For many years, efforts have been made to find new immunosuppressive drugs, more specific and potent, and with fewer side effects than steroids. Even cyclosporine-A did not meet these expectations. Antithymocyte globulins have been used both therapeutically in patients undergoing kidney transplant rejection or prophylactically. Unfortunately, no homogeneous results have been reported in the literature, probably because of lot-to-lot variations and reactivity with other blood components, such as human erythrocytes and/or platelets.

OKT3 PAN is a murine monoclonal antibody developed by Kung and colleagues.[1] It is secreted by a hybridoma produced by the procedure of Kohler and Millstein,[2] and it is directed against T3 antigen, a molecule present at the surface of almost all peripheral T lymphocytes.

Cosimi and colleagues[3] were the first to use OKT3 as an immunosuppressive agent in patients with an established acute renal rejection. Unlike these authors, we used OKT3 in the *prevention* of transplant rejection, in two different and consecutive randomized studies.

In the first study, our primary objective was to evaluate the ability of OKT3 to induce tolerance when it is administered as the sole immunosuppressive agent. Indeed, neither steroids nor azathioprine were given during OKT3 treatment, so that any observed effect could be attributed with no doubt to OKT3. It was initially planned to enroll 40 patients in this phase II randomized study. Informed consent was obtained from all patients. Only first cadaveric grafts were considered. Patients assigned to the control group were given azathioprine, 3 mg/kg/ day from the day before transplantation, and high-dose steroids: methylprednisolone, 1 g intravenously was administered during surgery, followed by oral prednisolone, 5 mg/kg/day, then progressively tapered to .25 mg/kg/day. Patients assigned to the experimental group were given OKT3 5 mg per day by intravenous route from the day before transplantation through day 13. No additional immunosuppressive drug nor steroids were given during this period of time. Azathioprine alone, 3 mg/kg/day, was introduced at day 14 and continued thereafter. In the case of a rejection, conventional treatment was started according to the same schedule as in the postsurgery period of the control group.

This study was discontinued before its completion for reasons that will be discussed later. Thus, only 13 patients were enrolled, six in the OKT3 group and seven in the steroid group. There were no differences between the two groups regarding age of patients, sex, duration of hemodialysis, total ischemia of the graft and HLA compatibility. All patients had received blood transfusions during the pretransplant period. However, patients in the control group received a slightly larger amount of blood. Nonresponders, according to the blood transfusion protocol used at Hôpital Necker, were also more numerous in this group than in the OKT3 group. Tolerance of OKT3 was generally good, except for the first injection, after which all patients experienced profuse diarrhea, fever, and chills. However, subsequent injections were well tolerated. There was no significant difference between the two groups concerning the occurrence of infections.

Why this protocol was discontinued before its completion is shown in Table 1: all patients in the OKT3 group developed an acute rejection episode, which occurred 12.8 ± 2.9 days after transplantation. Nevertheless, it is noteworthy that no rejection episode occurred within the first nine days even without additional immunosuppressive treatment. These data prove the strong immunosuppressive action of OKT3. As early as one hour after the first OKT3 injection, a dramatic and concomitant decrease of $T3^+$, $T4^+$ and $T8^+$ cells was observed. $T3^+$ cell level remained close to zero for up to 10 to 13 days posttransplant and then suddenly rose (Figure 1). Acute rejection was simultaneously observed.

Table 1
Protocol B81-052–OKT3/PAN, Starting January 1982

Groups	No.	ATN	1st Rejection Episode		Outcome		
			No.	Time Post Transplant (days)	Good Function	HDC	Dead
OKT3	6	5	6	12.8 ± 2.9	5	1	0
Control	8	3	3	33.3 ± 20.5	6	1	1

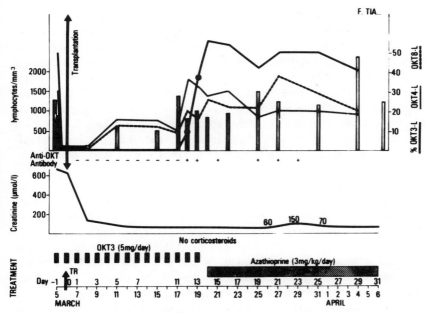

Figure 1 Typical example of the first-month course of patients on OKT3-Pan. The upper part of the figure represents blood level of OKT3$^+$ OKT4$^+$ and OKT8$^+$ lymphocytes. Columns represent the absolute number of lymphocytes per mm^3.

Therefore, the reappearance of T3$^+$ cells and the occurrence of rejection appear to be closely related. This sudden reappearance of T3$^+$ cells can be explained by two ways: 1) the discontinuation of OKT3; 2) in patients who were still receiving OKT3 when T3$^+$ cells reappeared, an immunization against the monoclonal antibody.

Indeed, in five of the six OKT3-treated patients, the serum level of OKT3 decreased during its administration, while anti-OKT3 antibodies appeared. Anti-OKT3 antibodies were mainly anti-idiotypic antibodies and antibodies directed against mouse IgG, as discussed by Dr. Chatenoud in this volume.

Early in the posttransplant period, while T3$^+$ cells were almost not detectable, T4$^+$ and T8$^+$ cells were present in the circulation (Figure 1). This indicates the appearance of OKT3$^-$4$^+$ and OKT3$^-$8$^+$ cells.

When these cells were incubated in vitro in the absence of OKT3, they reexpressed the OKT3-defined antigen, which was clearly detected as early as eight hours of incubation and was at its highest level after twenty hours. The reappearance of the OKT3-defined antigen was not prevented when cells had been irradiated with 1500 rads before setting up the culture, indicating that cell division was not a prerequisite. These data are best explained by the phenomenon of antigenic modulation, according to which the expression of a membrane antigen can be reversibly suppressed by the specific antibody. This phenomenon was demonstrated for the first time for the OKT3-defined antigen in Dr. Bach's laboratory in Hôpital Necker. In vitro, OKT3 induced capping of the OKT3-defined membrane antigen when lymphocytes, previously coated with antibody at 4C, were incubated for 30 minutes at 37C.

Thus, a new question is raised: which cells are accountable for rejection? $T3^+$ cells or modulating cells that previously appeared? In fact, one of us has shown that the mitogenic response of modulating cells, which is observed when they are cultivated in serum from individuals of the AB blood group, is completely abolished in the presence of autologous serum containing OKT3. This shows that, although potentially immunocompetent, modulating cells are functionally inactive as long as significant OKT3 levels are present in the serum. Nevertheless, this single in vitro test does not allow a definitive conclusion concerning the activity of modulating cells in vivo.

Thus, this first OKT3 trial showed that OKT3 is a powerful and well-tolerated immunosuppressive agent, which use is hampered by its immunogenicity. In order to abolish or to decrease anti-OKT3 antibody formation, we initiated a new protocol, which is still in progress, where OKT3 is associated with low-dose steroids and azathioprine.

Sixty patients are to be enrolled in this phase II study, randomly divided between three treatment groups. All patients receive azathioprine, 3 mg/kg/day, starting from the day before transplantation, and 1 g of IV methylprednisolone during surgery.

Patients of the first group (the CH group) are assigned to high-dose steroids and receive oral prednisolone, 5 mg/kg/day for five days, which is then progressively tapered to .25 mg/kg/day.

Patients of the second group (the CL group) are assigned to low-dose steroids and receive prednisolone, .25 mg/kg/day from day 1 through day 9, its dosage being increased to 1 mg/kg/day from day 10 through 14, and then progressively tapered to reach .25 mg/kg/day on day 30.

Patients of the third group (the EX group) receive steroids according to the same schedule as in the low-dose steroid group, and OKT3 5 mg/kg/day by IV injection from the day before transplantation through day 13. From day 14 through 30, OKT3 may be continued until $OKT3^+$ cells appear in the peripheral blood.

To date, 20 patients have been enrolled in this protocol. Therefore, it is not possible to state any definitive conclusion. However, when considering the 17 patients with a two-month follow-up, it appears that all six patients in the CL group experienced rejection within the first month, whereas rejection occurred in only two among the six OKT3-treated patients. Both these patients were immunized against the drug, with a reappearance of $T3^+$ cells.

Serum concentration of OKT3 was determined in patients from the two studies. In the first protocol, the drug disappeared from the serum before day 13, whereas its concentration remained the same during all the time of OKT3 administration when OKT3 was associated with low-dose steroids and azathioprine. This was due to a delayed appearance of anti-OKT3 antibodies of IgG type. Antibodies of the IgM type, which appeared some days before IgG, did not seem to induce the reappearance of circulating OKT3$^+$ cells.

The day of appearance of modulating cells was not modified by the associated immunosuppressive treatment. Indeed, modulating cells were detected in all six patients on days 5 to 7. Therefore, it is possible to assume that modulation of the OKT3-defined antigen by the monoclonal antibody never induced rejection.

In conclusion, it can be stated that OKT3 is a major immunosuppressive agent, with few side effects. However, it does not induce tolerance and its efficacy is restricted by its immunogenicity. This immunogenicity is delayed by association with conventional immunosuppressive treatment. OKT3 leads to modulation of the OKT3-defined membrane antigen, but modulation of the cells does not induce rejection.

The therapeutic use of monoclonal antibodies as immunosuppressive agents is still in its very beginning. Therefore, it is difficult to predict what place it will have in the treatment of transplant recipients. However, at least two ways of improvement can be foreseen: 1) characterization of new methods for suppressing OKT3s immunogenicity; 2) utilization of monoclonal antibodies directed against other T-cell receptors, namely the anti-T4 monoclonal antibody.

REFERENCES

1. Kung PC, Goldstein G, Reinherz EL, et al: Monoclonal antibodies defining distinctive human T cell surface antigens. *Science* 1979;206:347–349.
2. Kohler G, Millstein G: Continuous cultures of Fuse cells secreting antibody of predefined specificity. *Nature* 1975;265:495–497.
3. Cosimi AB, Colvin RB, Burton RC, et al: Use of monoclonal antibodies to T-Cell subsets for immunologic monitoring and treatment in recipients of renal allografts. *N Engl J Med* 1981;305:308.

9 Highly Successful Reversal of Renal Tranplant Rejection by Infusion of a Monocyte-Blast Cell Monoclonal Antibody (CBL1)

R. Billing, H. Takahashi, P. Terasaki,
Y. Iwaki, F. Hofmann

Previous studies have shown that an antiblast monocyte antibody, CBL1, could significantly prolong skin allograft survival in rhesus monkeys. It was postulated that this antibody might be eliminating activated clones of cells that were responsible for graft rejection. Here we describe the first clinical use of CBL1. Seventeen of 19 patients with severe kidney graft rejections had reversal of rejection episodes without observable adverse side effects. The patients were treated with daily infusions of 5 mg of CBL1. There was no significant change in blood lymphocyte or platelet count, nor any signs of fever or chills. Fifteen of the rejection episodes had failed steroid therapy, and in 12 cases the creatinine clearance was in excess of 7.8 mg/100 ml. If as postulated, CBL1 is eliminating activated clones of immune cells, CBL1 therapy may have widespread application in other diseases with an immunological etiology.

CBL1[1] was previously shown to significantly increase skin allograft survival in rhesus monkeys.[2,3] There were no apparent side effects, such as chills or fevers, or changes in peripheral blood cell counts. Therefore, CBL1 appeared to be a candidate for clinical trials. This report describes some aspects of the initial clinical trials of CBL1 in the treatment of kidney graft rejection. The results appear to be superior to those obtained with antibodies such as antithymocyte globulin (ATG) and pan-T monoclonals that are lytic for the whole population of peripheral blood T cells.[4] The differences in side effects, efficacy and long-term results may be due to the fact that CBL1 is not reacting with the majority of T cells, but only with activated cells involved in the rejection process.

METHODS

Kidney transplants from haplotype-matched living related donors were performed in 31 patients after donor-specific buffy coat transfusions given three times from 200 ml of donated blood. Since no rejection, or only mild rejections, were encountered in 20 patients, no monoclonal antibody (MCA) was administered to this group. Their one-year graft survival rate was 100%. The remaining 11 patients, with severe rejections for which the MCA was utilized, are the subjects of this report.

For 22 cadaver donor transplants, 15 kidneys from Caucasian donors were sent from the United States to Sendai. All patients received at least three transfusions. Since 14 patients had mild rejections, no MCA was used, and their one-year graft survival rate was 79%. We report here on eight patients with steroid-resistant or severe rejections treated with MCA.

Our standard protocol of antirejection treatment included intravenous methylprednisolone 10–20 mg/kg/day for three days; an increase in oral prednisolone to 3–4 mg/kg/day, and then reduced to 0.2 mg/kg/day; and 150 rads to the kidney on alternative days for a total of 450 rads. Rejection was diagnosed by the usual clinical and laboratory findings as well as by histopathological evaluation of transplant biopsies. A steroid-resistant rejection episode was defined as continuing elevation of serum creatinine three to five days after three 500 mg methylprednisolone pulses.

A description of the CBL1 antibody production and characteristics has been published.[1] This hybridoma was expanded in Senadi in BALB/c mice. The ascitic fluid from approximately 100 mice was collected, treated with ammonium sulfate, and safety-tested for pyrogen, sterility and toxicity. The IgM antibody had a 1:4000 titer in the original preparation. It was given intravenously (5 mg in 100 ml of saline) on nine successive days. There was no necessity to administer the antibody via a central vein.

RESULTS

The results are shown in Table 1. Nineteen patients rejection kidney transplants were treated with a nine-day course of CBL1. In 17 patients the rejection episodes were reversed. One of the failures had a plasma creatinine exceeding 10 mg/100 ml for several days prior to and during CBL1 treatment, and was probably treated too late. The only other treatment prior to CBL1 was with steroids or radiation to the kidney. Fifteen of the patients were considered to have steroid-resistant rejections, and 12 patients had peak serum creatinine clearance levels of over 7.8 mg/100 ml.

There were no observable side effects of the treatment. These included no infections, changes in blood cell counts, chills, or fevers. There were three subsequent rejections, one of which was reversed with a second treatment with CBL1 14 days after the first.

By immunoperoxidase binding studies, we have recently shown that the CBL1 antigen is present in the cytoplasm of resting peripheral blood lymphocytes but not on the surface of these cells. When lymphocytes are activated, the antigen appears on the cell surface, which allows them to be lysed in the presence of anti-body and complement.

DISCUSSION

CBL1 reacts only with blast cells such as PHA-activated T cells and a subpopulation of monocytes. Therefore, it has an entirely different specificity to previous forms of immunosuppression used to reverse graft rejection.

There are several important unique features of CBL1 reversal of kidney graft rejection that were not apparent with previous treatments with pan-T reagents.[4] One is that destruction of normal, resting, peripheral blood lymphocytes is not necessary for reversal of the rejection process. CBL1 appears to be much more specific for cells directly involved in the rejection than previous treatments, which relied on anti-lymphocyte effects. This feature is, of course, highly important with regard to the efficacy of the treatment and the lack of side effects. The second remarkable feature of CBL1 is that one course of treatment over nine days produced a permanent effect even in patients who had experienced severe rejections. Over 50% of the patients have now been followed for over 12 months. These lasting effects were not seen in patients treated with pan1T monoclonal antibody.[4]

CBL1 has now been used successfully at the University of California at San Diego in three kidney patients undergoing severe rejection episodes (J. Collins, R. Steiner, personal communication). However, in one other study, less successful results have been obtained immediately following antithymocyte globulin (ATGAM) treatment (R. Mendez, personal communication). A possible explanation for this is that the lytic effect of ATGAM on peripheral blood lymphocytes releases cytoplasmic soluble antigen, which blocks the subsequent effect of CBL1 on activated cells. Because previous batches of heterologous antilymphocyte serum (ALS) or ATG, such as ATGAM, contain lytic lymphocyte antibodies, it is most probable that their mode of action is *not* because they contain CBL1-like antibodies. Any CBL1-like antibodies would be blocked by the concomitant release of soluble antigen.

The possible modes of action of CBL1 have been discussed previously.[2,3] The most plausible theory is that clones of activated blast cells reactive against the allograft are being destroyed. The homing effect of mouse monoclonal antibodies to spleen may mean that these cells are also destroyed in situ as well as in the kidney itself.

The possible immunological-related disease that could be treated by this new approach are many and varied. We earnestly await future clinical studies that will determine whether this early optimism is justified.

Table 1
Results of Treatment of Steroid-Resistant Rejection with CBL1

No. of Case	LD or CD	No. of Mis-Matching	Blood Transfusion	Panel[§] Test (Tw%)	Days of Hemodialysis (PTD)[‖]	Day of Rejection (PTD)	Treated Rejection
1. YS	CD	A 2 B 2 DR 2	WBT* 20-30 unit	5	17	27	1st
2. EK	CD	A 1 B 2 DR 1	WBT 14 unit	5	47	28	1st
3. SH	CD	A 1 B 1 DR 2	WBT 10 unit	45	0	14	1st
4. MK	LD	1 haplo	DST[†] × 3	nt	0	7	1st
5. AS	CD	A2 B 1 DR 2	WBT 4 unit pooled-BCT	0	17	90	3rd
6. KS	LD	1 haplo	DST × 3	nt	10	6	1st
7. IA	CD 2nd	A 1 B 2 DR 1	WBT 8 unit pooled-BCT	3	14	190	3rd
8. YO	CD	A 2 B 2 DR 2	BCT 10 unit	41	0	26	1st
9. TA	LD	1 haplo	DST × 3	100	0	6	1st
10. KT	CD	A 1 B 2 DR 2	WBT* 10 unit	0	19	30	2nd
11. HW	LD	1 haplo	DST[†] × 3	81	23	4	1st
12. KK	LD	1 haplo	DST × 3	0	0	3	1st
13. KT	LD	1 haplo	DST × 3	nt	0	4	1st
14. MK	LD	1 haplo	DST × 3	0	0	9	1st
15. SF	LD	1 haplo	DST × 3	0	0	3	1st
16. HH	LD	1 haplo	DST × 3	nt	0	2	1st
17. FS	CD	A 2 B 2 DR 1	Pooled-BCT[‡]	0	0	182	5th
18. KA	LD	1 haplo	DST × 3	nt	26	12	1st
19. AK	LD	1 haplo	DST × 3	nt	0	36	2nd

*WBT: whole blood transfusion.
[†]DST: donor specific transfusion.
[‡]pooled-BCT: pooled buffy-coat transfusion.
[§]panel test: post-transfusion.
[‖]PTD: post-transplant day.

| Serum Creatinine (mg/100 ml) | | | Day of Treatment | | Days to Reversal | Efficacy | Outcome | | |
| | | | *Steroid* | | | | *Recurrent Rejection (mos after MCA)* | *Current Function* | *Status Pcr*** |
Prere-jection	*Peak*	*Post-MCA¶*	*Pulse (PTD)*	*MCA (PTD)*					
1.2	4.1	1.1	25,26	29–37	14	reversed	1	F	13 mos	3.8
3.3	8.9	2.3	27,28,29	34–42	28	reversed	0	IF	5 mos	–
1.4	3.2	1.6	13,15, 17,19	21–29	23	reversed	0	F	9 mos	3.3
1.0	2.8	1.4	7,8,9 10~24	12–20	11	reversed	0	F	7 mos	1.4
3.0	7.0	2.6	not done	96–104	27	reversed	0	F	15 mos	2.6
2.4	12.0	2.0	2,3	15–23	27	reversed	0	F	2 mos	2.0
1.4	3.7	2.1	172, 173, 174, 180	191–198	14	reversed	0	NIF	11 mos	–
5.8	11.3	7.0	2,3,4,5,6	28–36	–	not reversed	–	IF	45 day	–
1.0	10.8	2.6	2,4,5	9–17	60	reversed	0	F	4 mos	2.6
1.4	3.5	0.6	31,33	32–37	4	reversed	0	F	6 mos	0.6
5.0	11.5	1.5	2,9	8,10–13	14	reversed	0	F	9 mos	1.5
2.0	11.0	1.2	5,6,7	5–12	11	reversed	1	F	7 mos	2.7
2.0	6.0	1.2	2	6–14	12	reversed	0	F	5 mos	1.3
1.2	12.8	1.4	7,8,9,16	10–19	22	reversed	0	F	4 mos	1.4
1.7	7.8	1.1	3,7	7–16	20	reversed	1	F	8 mos	1.4
6.0	12.5	1.5	1,2,3	3–10	13	reversed	0	F	5 mos	1.7
3.0	4.3	2.3	189	189–197	8	reversed	0	F	11 mos	2.3
9.0	13.0	1.0	1,3	13–22	15	reversed	0	F	2 mos	1.0
3.5	10.5	4.0	36,38, 40,42	42–48	–	not reversed	0	F	2 mos	–

¶MCA: monoclonal antibody CBL1.
**Pcr: plasma creatinine (mg/100 ml).

REFERENCES

1. Billing R, Wells J, Zettel D, et al: Monoclonal and heteroantibody reacting with different antigens common to human blast cells and monocytes. *Hybridoma* 1982;1:303–311.
2. Billing R, Chatterjee S: Prolongation of skin allograft survival in monkeys treated with anti-Ia and antiblast/monocyte monoclonal antibodies. *Transplant Proc* 1983;15:649–650.
3. Chatterjee S, Bernoco D, Billing RJ: Treatment with anti-Ia and anti-blast/monocyte monoclonal antibodies can prolong skin allograft survival in non-human primates. *Hybridoma* 1982;1:369–377.
4. Cosimi AB, Burton RC, Colvin RB, et al: Treatment of acute renal allograft rejection with OKT3 monoclonal antibody. *Transplantation* 1981;32:535–539.

10 The Use of Monoclonal Antibodies Specific for T-Cell Subsets as Immunosuppressive Agents in Rhesus Monkeys

M. Jonker, P. Neuhaus, G. Goldstein

A large number of monoclonal antibodies (MCA) specific for antigens expressed on subpopulations of human lymphocytes has become available in the past few years. Apart from their value as reagents for studying lymphocyte differentiation and cellular interactions in the immune response, these MCAs will most likely replace antilymphocyte sera (ALS) as immunosuppressive agents in organ transplantation. The major advantage of MCAs over ALS is the selective kill of cell populations responsible for graft rejection, while the populations for other immune responses are not affected. Since many of the antihuman MCAs also react with lymphocytes of nonhuman primates, macaques are good subjects for testing of such reagents for efficacy and toxicity. Studies in cynomolgus monkeys have shown that OKT4, an MCA specific for human "helper T cells," can prolong kidney graft survival.[1] In the study reported here, the immunosuppressive effect of several antihuman MCAs was investigated in rhesus monkeys receiving skin or kidney allografts.

Injection of a MCA did not always result in the elimination of the T cells of the relevant subset from the circulation. Two other effects on the subsets were observed: "coating" and "modulation."[2,3] As can be seen in Table 1, the coating phenomenon occurred with three of the tested MCAs: OKT4 and OKT4A, both reactive with T4 cells, and B9.8 and B9 pool, MCAs reactive with T8 cells. An example of coating is given in Figure 1A. After injection of OKT4A, the relative numbers of T4 and T8 cells were monitored by using an indirect immunofluorescence technique and FACS analysis. No significant decrease in T4 cells was observed. However, an increase in numbers of cells stained with GM/F (goat antimouse Ig; FITC labeled) was found during the first 10 days of treatment, indicating that T4 cells coated with MCA were present in the circulation. After 10 to 13 days of treatment, the relative numbers of cells stained with GM/F returned to normal values, indicating that the T4 cells were no longer

92

coated with antibody in spite of continued treatment. This was the most likely due to the formation of antimouse IgG antibodies that neutralized the injected MCA. No significant change in the relative numbers of T8 cells was observed (after subtraction of the cells stained with GM/F). Interestingly, when OKT4 and OKT4A were injected simultaneously, the T4 cells were eliminated from the circulation (Figure 1B). Thus, when both the OKT4 and OKT4A antibody molecules are bound to the different antigenic determinants recognized by these antibodies, an efficient elimination of the lymphocytes by the lymphoreticuloendothelial system can occur.

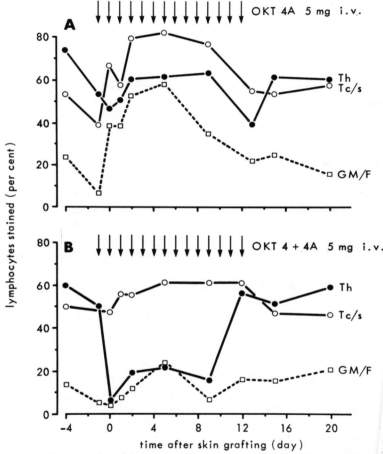

Figure 1 Effect of intravenous injection of OKT4 (**A**) and OKT4$^+$4A (**B**) MCAs on the relative numbers of T4 and T8 cells in peripheral blood lymphocytes. The vertical arrows indicate the timing of the injections. T4 and T8: relative number of "helper" and "cytotoxic/suppressor" T cells as defined by an indirect immunofluorescence test with OKT4A and OKT8A MCAs and FACS analysis. GM/F: relative number of cells stained with the second step antibody alone.

Table 1
Effect of Treatment of Rhesus Monkeys with Monoclonal Antibodies Against T-Cell Subsets

MCAs Used for Treatment	Immunoglobulin Class	Reactive Cell Population (as defined in humans)	Daily Antibody Dose	Effect on Relevant T-cell Subset	Skin Graft Survival (days)*
OKT4A	IgG2a	Helper T cells	5 mg per animal	Coating	16, 19
OKT4	IgG2b	Helper T cells	5 mg per animal	Coating	11.5, 18
OKT4 + OKT4A	IgG2b + IgG2a	Helper T cells	5 mg per animal	Elimination	13, 16
OKT8A	IgG2a	Cytotoxic/suppressor T cells	5 mg per animal	Slow elimination	10, 11
B9.8	IgG2a	Cytotoxic/suppressor T cells	0.5 mg/kg^{-1}	Coating	11.5, 12.5
B9 pool	IgG1,IgG2a,IgG3	Cytotoxic/suppressor T cells	0.5 mg/kg^{-1}	Coating or elimination	14, 15, 14
OKT11A	IgG2a	All periferal T cells	5 mg per animal	"Modulation"	13.5, 14
WT1	IgG2a	All periferal T cells	1.5 mg/kg^{-1}	"Modulation"	15, 17
42 untreated† control animals					10.3 ± (range: 8.5–13)

*Each number represents one skin graft survival time in a rhesus monkey.
†These were related and unrelated donor/recipient combinations differing for a single RhLA-A or B-locus.

Treatment with OKT11A or WT1 had an effect on the OKT11A or WT1-reactive cells that we have called "modulation." After treatment with these MCAs, the relative numbers of OKT11A and WT1-reactive cells decreased to background values, while those of T4 and T8 cells did not change. Since the T4 and T8 cells are contained in the OKT11A population, this indicates that the cells were not eliminated, but that the OKT11A antigen was internalized or shed from the cells (antigen modulation).

The daily injected MCA amount (Table 1, column 4) was in all instances sufficient to maintain significant MCA levels in the serum of treated monkeys until the next injection was given 24 hours later. However, after 10 to 13 days of treatment, the injected MCA was neutralized by antimouse IgG antibodies formed by the treated monkeys in all cases.

Skin graft survival time was significantly prolonged ($p < 0.05$, Mann-Whitney U-test) when the animals were treated with anti-Th MCAs (OKT4, OKT4A), irrespective of whether T4 cells were eliminated from the circulation or were just coated with anti-T4 antibody. These data suggest that the T4-cell population at least is important for skin allograft rejection. MCAs reactive with T8 cells (OKT8A, B9.8) injected separately did not prolong skin graft survival times. However, when a pool of antibodies reactive with T8 cells (B9 pool) was injected, a slight prolongation in skin graft survival time was observed ($p < 0.01$). The failure to observe prolongation of skin graft survival time with separate antibodies might be due to poor crossreactivity of these antibodies with rhesus cells. MCAs reactive with all T cells (OKT11A, WT1) resulted in a modest but significant prolongation ($p < 0.01$, Mann-Whitney U-test) of skin graft survival times. This is most likely because the cells responsible for graft rejection could not exert their immunological function when antigenic modulation occurred.

Since the injection of OKT4 and OKT4A resulted in skin graft survival times of up to 19 days, it was decided to test these antibodies for their capacity to prevent or reverse kidney allograft rejection. As the combination of the OKT4 and 4A antibodies had a more profound effect on the helper T cells, it was decided to use a one-to-one mixture of these two antibodies in these experiments. There were six experimental groups, all listed in Table 2. THe first group was an untreated control group. The second group received a three-week treatment course of 2.5 mg OKT4 mixed with 2.5 mg OKT4A intravenously daily, starting at two days before transplantation. The third group received a three week OKT4$^+$4A treatment course starting at five days after transplantation (early rejection treatment). All animals received an RhLA-A, B and DR mismatched kidney. Additional daily low doses of prehnisolone (1 mg/kg^{-1} and azathioprine (2 mg/kg^{-1}) were given, starting on the day of transplantation and continued for 45 days. Groups two and three both showed significant prolongation of kidney graft survival (Table 2). Thus, treatment with

Table 2
Effect of Various Treatment Regimes on Monkey Kidney Allografts

Group	Immunosuppression	Individual Survival Times	MST ± SE		
1. Controls	aza + pred*	9 9 10 10 11 12 13 14 14 17 22	12.8 ± 1.2	$p < 0.001$	$p < 0.05$
2. Pretreatment with OKT4 + 4A	aza + pred 5 mg OKT4+4A day $-2 \to 19$	14 30 31 37 46 53 59	38.6 ± 6.3		
3. Rejection treatment with OKT4 + 4A	aza + pred 5 mg OKT4 + 4A day $5 \to 26$	8 10 21 26 53 54 112	40.6 ± 14.9		
4. Transfused controls	aza + pred	9 10 11 12 12 13 13 19 22 29 32 32 34 41 43 43 44 53 53 56 56 61 75	33.6 ± 4.2 (48.8 ± 4.3)	n.s.	$p = 0.05$
5. Transfused pretreatment with OKT4 + 4A	aza + pred 5 mg OKT4 + 4A day $-2 \to 19$	10 18 26 41 50 59 92 92	48.5 ± 11.8		
6. Transfused rejection treatment with OKT4 + 4A	aza + pred 5 mg OKT4 + 4A for 21 days after serum creatinine $>200 \ \mu mol \times 1^{-1}$	35 44 45 60 67 71 107	61.3 ± 9.8		

*azathioprine 2 mg/kg^{-1} daily for 45 days; prednisolone 1 mg/kg^{-1} daily for 45 days.
O Control animals for group 6; MST of these animals in brackets.

OKT4$^+$4A antibody could prevent and reverse kidney allograft rejection.

Since most patients awaiting a kidney allograft are transfused prior to transplantation, it was important to see whether treatment with OKT4$^+$4A antibodies was also effective in transfused monkeys. Animals in groups 4, 5 and 6 (Table 2) received three pretransplant blood transfusions from random donors at two week intervals. The last transfusion was given at two to three weeks before transplantation. Blood donors shared no RhLA-A or B-locus antigens with the prospective kidney donors; therefore, there was no sensitization against these antigens. Pretransplant blood transfusions have a significantly favorable effect on kidney graft survival in rhesus monkeys,[4,5] as is found in man. No additional effect was observed when these transfused monkeys received OKT4$^+$4A treatment starting at two days before transplantation. It is possible that blood transfusions somehow render the OKT4$^+$ cells ineffective, so that elimination of these cells at the time of transplantation does not affect graft outcome. Whether these T4 cells are actively suppressed by another cell type, or are affected in some other way, remains to be established. Application of other antibodies reactive with other cell types may eventually give insight into the blood transfusion effect.

The last group (6) of transfused monkeys received OKT4$^+$4A treatment when the animals had serum creatinine level of 200 μmol/1^{-1} or higher. Only those that had a creatinine level of less than 200 μmol/1^{-1}

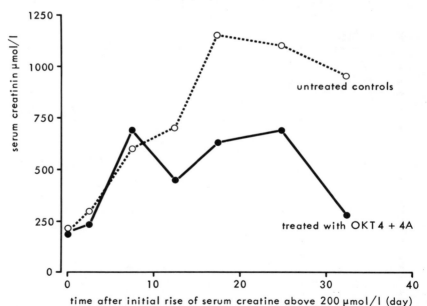

Figure 2 Median creatinine levels in transfused monkeys. Day 0 is day when the serum creatinine level was 200 μmol/1^{-1}.

during the first two weeks after transplantation were included in this group. The graft results of this group were compared with those of untreated transfused animals (from group 4) that also had a serum creatinine of less than 200 μmol/1^{-1} during the first two weeks after transplantation. Figure 2 shows that OKT4$^+$4A treated animals had lower serum creatinine levels than did the untreated controls. Three of seven OKT4$^+$4A treated animals showed a reversal to serum creatinine levels of less than 200 μmol/1^{-1} for a duration of one to three weeks, whereas only one of the two control animals showed a reversal to a serum of creatinine of less than 200 μmol/1^{-1} for five days. Also, graft survival after the initial increase in serum creatinine levels to 200 μmol/1^{-1} was significantly longer in the OKT4$^+$4A-treated group (34.7 days) as compared with the untreated group (19.1 days). Thus, in transfused monkeys, rejection treatment with OKT4$^+$4A antibody is possible. The T4 cells apparently do play a role in this "late" onset of rejection.

It can be concluded that monoclonal antibodies reactive with T cell subsets can be used as immunosuppressive agents in transplantation. Since these reagents are highly specific, it will be possible to select antibodies that will be very effective in preventing or reversing a rejection. Moreover, it will be possible in the rhesus monkey model to study the cells responsible for the blood transfusion effect in vivo. And this may then eventually lead to a better blood transfusion policy for patients awaiting kidney transplantation.

REFERENCES

1. Cosimi AB, Burton RC, Kung RC, et al: *Transplant Proc* 1981;13:499.
2. Jonker M, Malissen B, Mawas C: *Transplantation* 1983;35:374.
3. Jonker M, Goldstein G, Balner H: *Transplantation* 1983;35:521.
4. van Es AA, Marquet RL, Rood JJ, et al: *Lancet* 1977;1:506.
5. Borleffs JCC, Marquet RL, Balner H: *Transplantation* 1981;32:48.

11 A New Theory on the Mechanism of the Blood Transfusion Effect in Transplantation

P. I. Terasaki

The paradoxically beneficial effect of blood transfusions on subsequent kidney allografts is now explained by initially conceding that transfusions immunize the recipient. We then postulate that immunosuppression eliminates or inactivates the immunoblastic cells that result as a secondary response to the graft. The reason immunized patients have better graft survival than nonimmunized patients is attributed to the fact that immunosuppression conventionally is given in a high dose soon after transplantation, thus being more ideally timed for an early rejection rather than a rejection that occurs in one to two weeks.

THE HYPOTHESIS

The mechanisms by which transfusions produce their beneficial effect remain largely unknown despite considerable investigative efforts in the past 10 years. We wish to advance a new hypothesis on the mechanisms responsible for the transfusion effect. We propose that the primary function of transfusions is to *immunize* recipients. Subsequent transplantation of a kidney elicits an anamnestic response. If the patient is then treated with high doses of immunosuppression, the reactive cells will be killed or inactivated. Loss of these reactive clones of cells then leaves the recipient in a nonresponsive state against the specific antigens. If the preimmunization step is omitted, transplanted kidneys would not induce a secondary response and the timing of high-dose immunosuppression at transplantation becomes premature. When the real rejection occurs, drugs cannot again be increased to high levels since the patient has already received the maximum tolerable dose. Therefore, the critical difference between a transfused and nontransfused patient is in the timing of rejection in relation to maximal immunosuppression. Since most centers use the highest dose at the time of transplantation, preimmunization by transfusions would fit the immunosuppression protocol better than no prior sensitization. In other words, since immunosuppression is provided at the maximum dose at transplantation, this regimen happens to be more appropriate for preimmunized, transfused patients than nonsensitized patients.

99

In defense of the hypothesis, we will consider the three main components: transfusions immunize; immunosuppression is necessary; and immunosuppression deletes reactive clones.

1. Immunization results from transfusions. Most of the data that has accrued on transfusions has been consistent with the simple hypothesis that transfusions actually immunize patients.

a. The most immunogenic cells, that is, the white cells, probably produce the transfusion effect.[1] Removal of white cells results in the loss of the transfusion effect.[2] Any treatment, such as freezing, that might decrease the transplantation antigens appears to decrease the transfusion effect.[3] Platelets that have HLA antigens also produce the transfusion effect.[4]

b. Most evidence indicates that transfusions are more effective when given before transplantation.[5,6] Transfusions given at least one month up to one year before transplantation are effective. In contrast, transfusions given at surgery have a weaker effect.

c. Multiple transfusions produce a greater transfusion effect.[7,8] Although a single transfusion is better than none,[2] additional transfusions, to about 10–15 units, progressively improve graft outcome.[3]

d. If the same donor is used for transfusion and for the kidney transplant, transplants are successful.[9] In experimental mice transfused and then treated with antilymphocyte serum (ALS), blood transfusions from specific donor strains are more effective than from unrelated strains.[10]

e. Following blood transfusions, about one-third of the patients developed cytotoxic antibodies, demonstrating that they were immunized.[11] Even in those patients who showed evidence of being immunized by having cytotoxic antibodies, the beneficial transfusion effect was obtained.[3,12-14] It is necessary to avoid transplantation only across a positive crossmatch. Even donors against whom the recipient had been latently sensitized in the past can be utilized.[15] This also indicates that prior immunization does not affect transplantability.

From the foregoing, the unavoidable conclusion is that transfusions immunize. Despite the immunization, the graft survival rate is high.

2. Immunization followed by immunosuppression is necessary to achieve the salutary effect of transfusion.

a. In experimental canine renal allografts, azathioprine and prednisone were essential for the transfusion effect to manifest itself. In Niessen et al's experiments, none of the transfused dogs had kidney graft survival for more than 28 days, whereas among dogs receiving transfusions plus immunosuppression, 80% of the grafts survived more than 28 days.[16] In dogs receiving immunosuppression alone, 44% of the grafts survived 28 days. Thus, transfusion or immunosuppression alone was ineffective whereas, combined, graft prolongation was obtained.

In 1969 Wilson et al reported similar results when they treated dogs with spleen antigens.[17] The mean kidney graft survival time was 144 days for those dogs receiving the antigen with azathioprine and prednisone compared with 90 days for dogs treated with immunosuppression alone, and seven days for those given antigens alone.

Many experiments indicate that azathioprine and prednisone together with transfusions produce extended graft survival.[18-20] Similarly, cyclosporine is also potentiated by blood transfusions.[21-23] The effect of ALS is markedly potentiated by blood transfusions when transfusions or antigens are injected first, and then the animals are treated with ALS.[24,25]

Although there are some experiments indicating that the transfusion effect can be obtained without immunosuppression,[26] the effect is a rather weak one in rat and dog kidney transplants.[27,28] We postulate that endogenous steroids released during the stress of the operation in these animals account for autoimmunosuppression. There is abundant evidence indicating that ACTH is markedly increased during periods of surgical stress.[29]

3. Immunosuppression either kills or inactivates clones that react against the graft.

Steroids have had a marked effect on lymphocytes.[30] When injected, they kill lymphocytes and cause involution of lymphoid organs. It is postulated that the clones that are stimulated by the immunization are then inactivated by the steroids. Other immunosuppressants may not necessarily kill lymphoid cells, but they may all act by inhibiting further mitosis of the reactive cells. Brent and Medawar proposed that sensitization consists mainly of a quantitative increase in numbers of reactive cells.[31] They postulated that immunosuppressants stop the further multiplication of cells. If the immunosuppressants hold the cells in check, the graft can survive, although it may be chronically attacked by a few surviving cells. We assume that with current immunosuppression, reactive clones are not completely eliminated, necessitating continuous treatment. This accounts for positive MLC reactions against donors in long-surviving donor recipient pairs.

The commonly encountered phenomenon of rejection reversal may consist of the destruction of reactive cells by immunosuppression. Once this is accomplished, the patient can then be free of further rejections.

Transfusions followed by immunosuppression given even *before*

102

transplantation would also be expected to suppress the reactive clones. In fact, this regimen has resulted in high graft survival rates in experimental dog transplants[32,33] and clinical grafts.[34]

CONSEQUENCES OF THE HYPOTHESIS

If transfusions serve to immunize, immunization can be accomplished more effectively than by transfusions. For example, rather than frequently transfusing whole blood, a "transplant antigen vaccine" composed of antigens from many donors might be administered. To kill the reacting clones of cells, monoclonal antibodies directed against antigens unique to activated cells, as used recently to reverse transplant rejection,[35] may be ideal. The monoclonal antibody to blast cells did not reduce peripheral blood lymphocyte counts in any of the 19 patients treated. As an added feature, according to the hypothesis, sensitized patients could be reimmunized and treated to remove the specifically reactive cells.

Once a patient is "decloned," he can then proceed to the second transplantation phase. In this way, the two risk factors, immunosuppression and surgical trauma, are decoupled into different time periods. Currently, since both surgery and immunosuppression occur simultaneously, the patient is subjected to a double risk. Because inactivation of clones against transplantation antigens would not affect lymphoid cells reactive against other antigens, this approach opens the door to the long-sought specific immunosuppression against transplant antigens.

REFERENCES

1. Opelz G, Terasaki PI: Improvement of kidney graft survival with increased numbers of transfusions. *N Engl J Med* 1978; 299:799–803.
2. Persijn GG, Cohen B, Lansbergen Q, et al: Retrospective and prospective studies on the effect of blood transfusions in renal transplantation in the Netherlands. *Transplantation* 1979;28:396–401.
3. Horimi T, Terasaki PI, Chia D, et al: Factors influencing the paradoxical effect of transfusions on kidney transplants. *Transplantation* 1983;35:320–323.
4. Borleffs JCC, Neuhaus P, van Rood JJ, et al: Platelet transfusions improve kidney allograft survival in Rhesus monkeys without inducing cytotoxic antibodies. *Lancet* 1982;1:1117–1118.
5. Opelz G, Terasaki PI. Importance of preoperative (not peroperative) transfusions for cadaver kidney transplants. *Transplantation* 1981;31:106–108.
6. Hourmant M, Soulillou JP, Bui-Quang D: Beneficial effect of blood transfusion. Role of the time interval between the last transfusion and transplantation. *Transplantation* 1979;28:40–43.
7. Opelz G, Graver B, Terasaki PI: Induction of high kidney graft survival rate by multiple transfusions. *Lancet* 1981;1:1223–1225.
8. Fehrman I: Pretransplant blood transfusions and related kidney allograft survival. *Transplantation* 1982;34:46–49.

9. Salvatierra O Jr, Iwaki Y, Vincenti F, et al: Incidence, characteristics, and outcome of recipients sensitized after donor-specific blood transfusions. *Transplantation* 1981;32:528–531.
10. Okazaki H, Maki T, Wood M, et al: Effect of a single transfusion of donor-specific and nonspecific blood on skin allograft survival in mice. *Transplantation* 1980;30:421–424.
11. Opelz G, Graver B, Mickey MR, et al: Lymphocytotoxic antibody responses to transfusions in potential kidney transplant recipients. *Transplantation* 1981;32:177–183.
12. Werner-Fevre C, Jeannet M, Harder F, et al: Blood transfusions, cytotoxic antibodies, and kidney graft survival. *Transplantation* 1979;28:343–346.
13. Feduska NJ, Vincenti F, Amend WJ Jr, et al: Do blood transfusions enhance the possibility of a compatible transplant? *Transplantation* 1979;27:35–38.
14. Sanfilippo F, Vaughn WK, Bollinger RR, et al: The relationship of transfusion and presensitization with graft and patient survival. *Transplant Proc* 1982;14:287–289.
15. Cardella CJ, Falk JA, Nicholson MJ, et al: Successful renal transplantation in patients with T-cell reactivity to donor. *Lancet* 1982;2:1240–1243.
16. Niessen GJCM, Obertop H, Bijnen AB, et al: Expression of beneficial blood transfusion effect in dogs is dependent upon immunosuppressants used. *Transplant Proc* 1982;14:400–402.
17. Wilson RE, Rippin A, Dagher RK, et al: Prolonged canine renal allograft survival after pretreatment with solubilized antigen. *Transplantation* 1969;7: 360–371.
18. Obertop H, Bijnen AB, Vriesendorp HM, et al: Prolongation of renal allograft survival in DLA tissue-typed beagles after third-party blood transfusions and immunosuppressive treatment. *Transplantation* 1978;26:255–259.
19. Fabre JW, Bishop M, Sen T, et al: A study of three protocols of blood transfusion before renal transplantation in the dog. *Transplantation* 1978;26:94–98.
20. van Es AA, Marquet RL, van Rood JJ, et al: Blood transfusions induce prolonged kidney allograft survival in Rhesus monkeys. *Lancet* 1977;1:506–509.
21. Borleffs JCC, de By-Aghai Z, Marquet RL: Beneficial influence of cyclosporin A and standard immunosuppression on kidney graft survival in transfused Rhesus monkeys. *Transplantation* 1981;32:161–162.
22. Miller CM, Martinelli GP, Racelis D, et al: Prolongation of rat cardiac allografts by pretransplant administration of blood transfusions and cyclosporin A. *Transplantation* 1982;33:335–337.
23. Borel JF, Feurer C, Magnee C, et al: Effects of the new antilymphocytic peptide cyclosporin A in animals. *Immunology* 1977;32:1017–1025.
24. Brent L, Hansen JA, Kilshaw PJ, et al: Specific unresponsiveness to skin allografts in mice. I. Properties of tissue extracts and their synergistic effect with anti-lymphocytic serum. *Transplantation* 1973;15:160–171.
25. Okazaki H, Maki T, Wood ML, et al: Prolongation of skin allograft survival in H-2 K and I region-incompatible mice by pretransplant blood transfusion. *Transplantation* 1981;32:111–115.
26. Halasz NA, Orloff MJ, Hirose F: Increased survival of renal homografts in dogs after injection of graft donor blood. *Transplantation* 1964;2:453–458.
27. Marquet RL, Heystek GA, Tinbergen WJ: Specific inhibition of organ allograft rejection by donor blood. *Transplant Proc* 1971;3:708–710.
28. Fabre JW, Morris PJ: The effect of donor strain blood pretreatment on renal allograft rejection in rats. *Transplantation* 1972;14:608–617.
29. Selye H: *Stress*. Montreal, Acta, Inc., 1951.
30. White A: Influence of endocrine secretions on the structure and function of

lymphoid tissue. *The Harvey Lectures 1947–48*. Springfield, Ill, Charles C. Thomas, 1950.

31. Brent L, Medawar P: Quantitative studies on tissue transplantation immunity. VII. The normal lymphocyte transfer reaction. *Proc R Soc Lond (Biol)* 1966;165:281–307.

32. Van der Linden CJ, Buurman WA, et al: Effect of blood transfusions on canine renal allograft survival. *Transplantation* 1982;33:400–402.

33. Iwaki Y, Kinukawa T, Terasaki PI, et al: Donor-specific transfusion from unrelated dogs and evidence against the selection mechanism. *Transplant Proc* 1983;15:979–984.

34. Anderson CB, Sicard GA, Etheredge EE: Pretreatment of renal allograft recipients with azathioprine and donor-specific blood products. *Surgery* 1982;92:315.

35. Takahashi H, Okazaki H, Terasaki PI, et al: Reversal of transplant rejection by monoclonal antiblast antibody. *Lancet*, in press.

12 Diversity of the Immunization Against the Monoclonal Antibody OKT3 in Renal Allograft Recipients

L. Chatenoud, M.F. Baudrihaye,
H. Kreis, J.F. Bach

Monoclonal antibodies produced by murine hybridomas and directed against human T cells are now widely used as immunosuppressive agents in clinical transplantation.[1,2] Our experience is centered on the prophylactic use of the OKT3 antibody (ORTHO Pharmaceutical Corp., Raritan, NJ) administered alone (5 mg/day IV for 13 days),[2] or in association with conventional immunosuppressants (OKT3 5 mg/day, IV for 30 days, corticosteroids 0.25 mg/kg/day, azathioprine 3 mg/kg/day).

Six patients were treated with OKT3 alone. In all these patients a complete disappearance of all peripheral T cells was observed soon after the first injection. This T-cell depletion demonstrated the high immunosuppressive potency of the murine antibody.[2] Importantly, however, in all patients T cells reappeared in the circulation by the second and the fifth day posttreatment. These cells were T cells, as assessed by the OKT4 or OKT8 reactivity. They were abnormal, though, since they lacked OKT3 reactivity because of in vivo antigenic modulation of the OKT3 defined membrane antigen.[2] All details concerning in vivo and in vitro characteristics of these modulated cells, as well as the practical and theoretical relevance of the modulation phenomenon itself, have been extensively described elsewhere.[2,3]

Another major escape mechanism from OKT3 treatment was the rapid and intense immunization observed in five out of the six patients studied. In most subjects, significant proportions of circulating IgG anti-OKT3 antibodies, detected by ELISA, appeared by day 9-10 post treatment. These antibodies completely neutralized the immunosuppressive effect of the injected monoclonal, as shown by the disappearance of free circulating OKT3 (detected by ELISA) and the reappearance of peripheral OKT3+ cells before the cessation of treatment.[2] A detailed analysis of the anti-OKT3 antibody specificity revealed their high heterogeneity.

These studies used total sera as well as purified fractions obtained by two purification steps comprising ammonium sulfate precipitation, followed by passage through a Sepharose 4B column (Pharmacia, Uppsala, Sweden) coupled to UPC 10, a BALB/c myeloma protein of the IgG2a subclass (like OKT3). Sera and fractions were tested using the ELISA assay in which the complete OKT3 molecule as well as its F(ab)$'_2$ and Fab fragments were employed to coat the microplates. This method allows a simple detection of anti-OKT3 antibodies that react with the variable portion of the OKT3 molecule, presumably anti-idiotype antibodies (Table 1).

In parallel to these ELISA assays, two immunofluorescence tests were carried out to analyze the capacity of anti-OKT3 antibodies: 1) to bind to normal T cells previously coated with OKT3, their fragments, and the OKT8 control monoclonal, also of the IgG2a class (Table 2); 2) to inhibit the binding of OKT3, its fragments, and OKT8 to normal T cells (Table 3).

These studies showed, in four of the six patients treated with OKT3 alone, the existence of two main families of antibodies.

The first one comprised antimouse immunoglobulins that bound to the Seph 4B-UPC 10 column as well as to OKT3 or OKT8-coated T cells, but not T lymphocytes coated with the F(ab)$'_2$ or Fab fragments of OKT3 (Table 2). These antibodies did not inhibit the binding of OKT3, nor of its fragments, nor of OKT8 to normal T cells (Table 3).

The second category of antibodies showed anti-idiotypic specificity. Such antibodies were not retained on the Seph 4B-UPC 10 column and bound to normal T cells coated with either OKT3 or its fragments (Table 2). They completely inhibited the binding of OKT3 or F(ab)$'_2$ fragments to normal T cells, while not interfering with OKT8 binding to its target (Table 3).

Interestingly, one of the six patients showed a unique, very restricted response: only antimouse antibodies could be detected while the anti-idiotype component of the response was absent.

Table 1
Immunization Pattern of Patients Treated with OKT3
Alone as Detected by the ELISA Assay

Days Post Transplant	IgG Antibodies Reacting with		
	OKT3	OKT3 F(ab)$'_2$	OKT3 Fab
Before grafting	−	−	−
Day 7	−	−	−
Day 12	+ + +	+ +	−
Day 15	+ + +	+ + +	+ + +
Day 20	+ + +	+ + +	+ + +
Day 23	+ + +	+ + +	+ + +
Day 42	+ + +	+ + +	+ + +

Table 2
Immunofluorescence Assay to Define the Binding Capacity
of Purified Anti-OKT3 Antibodies

	% Cells Labeled with GAM-FITC*	% Doubly Labeled Cells GAM-FITC and GAHu-TRITC*
+ OKT3 + F_1†	84	84
+ OKT8 + F_1	14	4
+ OKT3 F(ab)$'_2$ + F_1	80	80
+ OKT3 Fab + F_1	50	22
+ OKT3 + F_2‡	80	80
+ OKT8 + F_2	14	14
+ OKT3 F(ab)$'_2$ + F_2	80	0

*In this assay, normal T cells were first incubated for 30 minutes at 4 C with OKT3 or fragments or OKT8, then washed and incubated for 30 minutes at 4 C with the purified antibody fractions. The cells were then washed again and incubated with a mixture of fluoresceinated goat antimouse antiserum (GAM-FITC) and rhodamine-labeled goat antihuman light chain antiserum (GAHu-TRITC).
†F_1 = fraction containing anti-OKT3 antibodies not retained on Seph 4B-UPC 10 column: anti-idiotypic antibodies.
‡F_2 = fraction containing anti-OKT3 antibodies that bound the Seph 4B-UPC 10 column: antimouse antibodies.

Table 3
Immunofluorescence Assay to Define the Inhibitory Capacity
of Purified Anti-OKT3 Antibodies

	% Cells Labeled with GAM-FITC*	% Doubly Labeled Cells: GAM-FITC and GAHu-TRITC*
+ OKT3 + F_1†	0	0
+ OKT8 + F_1	25	3
+ OKT3 − F(ab)$'_2$ + F_1	0	0
+ OKT3 + F_2‡	87	67
+ OKT8 + F_2	22	22
+ OKT3 − F(ab)$'_2$ + F_2	96	0

*In this assay the purified antibody fractions were first incubated with the antibodies OKT3 (or its fragments) or OKT8 for 30 minutes at 4 C; then normal T cells were added and incubated with the mixture for 30 minutes at 4 C. The cells were then washed and incubated again at 4 C for 30 minutes with a mixture of fluoresceinated goat antimouse antiserum (GAM-FITC) and rhodamine-labeled goat antihuman light chain antiserum (GAHu-TRITC).
†F_1 = fraction containing anti-OKT3 antibodies not retained on Seph 4B-UPC 10 column: anti-idiotypic antibodies.
‡F_2 = fraction containing anti-OKT3 antibodies that bound the Seph 4B-UPC 10 column: antimouse antibodies.

108

The intense immunization obtained in most patients treated with OKT3 alone and its subsequent deleterious effect on the murine antibody-induced immunosuppression, prompted us to modify the therapeutical protocol by adding corticosteroids and azathioprine to OKT3. By now, five patients were treated in that way. Their immunization pattern is presented in Table 4. The appearance of anti-OKT3 antibodies in most of these subjects was clearly delayed in comparison to patients treated with OKT3 alone. In addition, even when present, the anti-OKT3 antibodies detected in those patients showed significantly lower titer than those encountered in the subjects treated with OKT3 alone. Moreover, during the 30 days of the OKT3 treatment, all these patients, but one, exhibited significant titer of free-circulating OKT3 in their serum. This finding implies that the IgM anti-OKT3 antibodies present in patients SOU, MOR, ARE, and VAN had a low affinity, insufficient to neutralize the injected OKT3 as IgG antibodies do. Because of this low affinity, it was difficult to analyze the fine specificity of these IgM antibodies. However, in subjects DEB and SOU, the IgG anti-OKT3 antibodies also present exhibited antimouse, as well as anti-idiotype reactivity.

In conclusion, OKT3, as other monoclonal antibodies, induces a variety of antimouse Ig antibodies. These antibodies may be specific of mouse determinants, sometimes of well-defined isotype, as we observed in one patient who showed a restricted response against the IgG2a isotype. In other cases, they react exclusively with the variable portion, presumably with the idiotypic determinants. The presence of these antibodies may negate the immunosuppressive activity of OKT3. Importantly, the addition of low doses of conventional immunosuppressive treatment (steroids and azathioprine) delays very significantly the onset of ant-Ig sensitization, and favors the predominant appearance of IgM antibodies rather

Table 4
Monitoring of Circulating Anti-OKT3 Antibodies in Patients Treated with OKT3 + Corticosteroids + Azathioprine

DEB*	IgM detected from day 9 post treatment IgG detected from day 7 post treatment
SOU	IgM detected from day 21 to day 33 post treatment IgG detected from day 30 to day 60 post treatment
MOR	IgM detected from day 19 to day 90 post treatment IgG not detected
ARE	IgM detected from day 10 to day 35 post treatment IgG not detected
VAN	IgM detected from day 10 to day 35 post treatment

*This patient exhibited a slightly positive OKT3 skin test before the first injection, that may, perhaps, explain his strong reaction to the xenogenic antibody.
For the dosages, we used a specific ELISA assay, already described.

than the IgG antibodies found when OKT3 is administered alone. These data are central to the practical use of OKT3 as a therapeutic immunosuppressant. They may guide future trials of tolerance induction to mouse immunoglobulins.

REFERENCES

1. Cosimi AB, Colvin RB, Burton RC, et al: Use of monoclonal antibodies to T-cell subsets for immunologic monitoring and treatment in recipients of renal allografts. *N Engl J Med* 1981;305:308.
2. Chatenoud L, Baudrihaye MF, Kreis H, et al: Human in vivo antigenic modulation induced by the anti-T cell OKT3 monoclonal antibody. *Eur J Immunol* 1982:12:979.
3. Chatenoud L, Bach JF: Antigenic modulation, a major effector mechanism of antibody action. New roles in viral and autoimmune disease pathogenesis and in the escape from tumors and from the therapeutic action of monoclonal antibodies. *Immunology Today* (in press).

13 Depletion of T Cells from Human Bone Marrow with Monoclonal Antibody CT-2 and Complement for Prevention of Graft versus Host Disease in Allogenic Histocompatible and Nonhistocompatible Bone Marrow Transplantation

M.E. Trigg, M.J. Bozdech, R. Billing, P.M. Sondel, R. Hong, S.D. Horowitz, R. Exten, J.L. Finlay, R. Moen, W. Longo, C. Erickson, A. Peterson

Eight patients received T lymphocyte-depleted histocompatible bone marrow and 15 patients received T lymphocyte-depleted nonhistocompatible bone marrow. All eight patients receiving matched bone marrow quickly engrafted without severe graft vs. host disease (GvHD). None of the eight received anti-GvHD prophylaxis medications. Two of these eight patients are currently alive. Nonengraftment and severe GvHD were problems seen in some of the patients given the histoincompatible bone marrow. Four of these 15 patients are currently alive. T lymphocyte-depleted marrow is a promising form of treatment in both histocompatible and histoincompatible bone marrow transplants.

Bone marrow transplantation (BMT) has an established place in the management and treatment of patients with acute leukemias, aplastic anemia, immunodeficiency syndromes, and chronic myelogenous leukemia.[1-11] However, its widespread use has been limited by two major problems—the lack of histocompatible donors for many patients whose disease might yield to intensive chemoradiotherapy; and the high incidence of acute graft-versus-host disease (GvHD), limiting the availability of BMT to centers with the personnel and expertise to care for the patient with GvHD.[12-15]

Many different chemotherapeutic and immunomodulating agents have been used to diminish or prevent GvHD in the HLA-MLC compatible transplants as well as in mismatched transplants.[15-25] Despite these measures, adverse effects are frequent and none of these drugs or antibody preparations have appeared to significantly decrease the incidence of GvHD (Grade 2-4) below that of 40–50%.[15] A more recent technique, helpful in preventing GvHD in mouse transplant models when a bone marrow graft was histoincompatible,[26] involves depleting immunocompetent T lymphocytes from donor bone marrrow using antibodies to the T lymphocytes with and without complement. Several centers have treated donor bone marrow in vitro with OKT3 in the matched BMT setting,[20,21] or have used lectin binding as a physical means of depleting T lymphocytes.[22,23] However, except for one series from London where the incidence of acute GvHD was 18%,[20] the results of these manipulations have not been encouraging in treating aplastic anemia and hematologic malignancy, although three patients with combined immunodeficiency significantly benefited from lectin-separated marrow transplants from parents.[22] A single report of monoclonal-antibody treatment of maternal marrow suggested engraftment with immunocompetent cells was possible.[19] Of interest in this case was the occurrence of extremely severe GvHD. However, in vivo administration of the monoclonal antibody controlled the symptomatology.

We report our results treating 23 patients who had either acute leukemia, chronic myelogenous leukemia (CML), aplastic anemia (AA), immunodeficiency syndromes or non-Hodgkin's lymphoma.

MATERIALS AND METHODS

Patients

Clinical data for the 23 patients are given in Table 1. Three patients had AA; six patients had acute lymphocytic leukemia (ALL) in first, second, or third remission; two patients had chronic phase CML; one child had juvenile CML in accelerated phase; one adult had relapsed T-cell lymphoma; four children had severe combined immunodeficiency; one child had Wiskott-Aldrich syndrome; and five patients had acute myeloid leukemias (AML) in first or second remission, except for patient 037-23, who had an M2A marrow pre-BMT. All patients were accepted for BMT because of the poor prognosis associated with their diseases, and all gave written informed consent for BMT and for the donor bone marrow to be depleted of T lymphocytes.

Fifteen patients were given bone marrow from HLA-MLC mismatched donors with various degrees of phenotypic identity, and all these except for patient 026-12 had positive MLC reactivity. All the donors for the mismatched transplants, except in case 036-22, were related to the recipients. Eight patients were given HLA-MLC identical bone marrow from sibling donors.

None of the patients receiving sibling-matched (HLA A, B, C, D identical and MLC nonreactive) bone marrow received any methotrexate or other medication to prevent graft rejection or GvHD; however, patient 033-19, with AA, received antithymocyte globulin (ATG) and prednisone after her second transplant to prevent rejection. Five of the 15 mismatched patients received cyclophosphamide (2.5–7.5 mg/kg every other day) and prednisone (1 mg/kg/day) post transplant to prevent graft rejection and GvHD (patients 025-11, 031-17, 035-21, 036-22, and 037-23). None of the other 10 patients receiving mismatched marrow were given medications post transplant to prevent GvHD or graft rejection.

BMT Conditioning

The conditioning regimens used for the 23 patients are detailed in Table 1.

Bone Marrow Harvest

Bone marrow was aspirated from the anterior and posterior iliac crests of the anesthetized donor. The bone marrow was mixed with RPMI 1640 with glutamine (GIBCO, Grand Island, NY) plus heparin 50 units/ml of media. The aspirated volumes ranged from 300 ml to 1500 ml and were placed into 600 ml Fenwal blood bags.

T-Cell Depletion of Bone Marrow

CT-2 is an IgM mouse monoclonal antibody to the E-rosette receptor on T lymphocytes, and has been found to be non-toxic to myeloid and erythroid precursors when normal bone marrow is treated in the presence of rabbit complement. Patterns of reactivity of CT-2 are given in Table 2. Baby rabbit serum (Pel Freeze, Arkansas) is used as the source of complement. Each lot of complement used for individual donor marrow treatment is screened on a sample of donor marrow two to four weeks before the scheduled transplant.

The Fenwal bags of bone marrow are centrifuged to remove the plasma and fat and the buffy coat cells are then concentrated. CT-2 antibody is added to the buffy coat cells and, following a 30 minute incubation, baby rabbit serum is added. After an additional 60 minute incubation, the excess antibody and complement are removed; the bone marrow cells are resuspended in donor plasma and infused into the recipients over a two- to three-hour period through the central venous catheter. Details

114

Table 1
Clinical Data on the 23 Patients Described in This Report Who Underwent BMT with T-Lymphocyte Depleted Marrow

UPN	Dx	Age-Sex	Donor	HLA-MLC	Disease Status Pre-BMT	Preparative Regimen (initial regimen)
021-01	ALL	8 M	S	match	2nd remission	C,TBI-1
016-02	APML	19 M	S	match	1st remission	C,TBI-2
017-03	CML-j	2 F	Fa	A,B,C haplo; MLC+	accelerated phase	C,A-1,TBI-1
018-04	APML	27 M	S	B haplo; MLC+	1st remission	C,TBI-2
019-05	ALL	29 M	S	match	2nd remission	N,TBI-2
020-06	ALL	8 M	S × 2 Fa × 1	HLA match; MLC+ A,B,C haplo; MLC+	3rd remission	C,TBI-1
021-07	CML	26 M	B	match	1st chronic phase	C,TBI-2
022-08	AML	29 F	B × 2	A,B,C haplo; MLC+	3rd remission	C,A-2,TBI-2
023-09	SCID	1 M	Fa × 2	A,B,C haplo; MLC+	N/A	none for BMT #1 B,C* for BMT #2
024-10	ALL	39 F	S	HLA match; MLC+	1st remission	C,TBI-2

ID	Diagnosis	Age/Sex	Donor	Match/MLC	Disease status	Regimen
025-11	AA	22 M	B × 2	A,B,C haplo; MLC+	N/A	C*,TBI-3
026-12	WA	3 mos M	Fa	A haplo; MLC-	N/A	B,C*
027-13	SCID	4 M	Fa	A,B,C haplo; MLC+	N/A	none
028-14	SCID	1 M	F	A,B,C haplo; MLC+	N/A	none
029-15	CML	22 M	B	match	1st chronic phase	C,TBI-2
030-16	ALL	17 F	S	match	3rd remission	D,C,TBI-1
031-17	AML	26 F	B	A,B haplo; MLC+	3rd remission	C,TBI-2
032-18	ALL	26 F	S	match	1st remission	C,TBI-2
033-19	AA	10 F	S × 2	match	N/A	C*,TBI-3
034-20	SCID	4 M	Fa	B haplo; MLC+	N/A	B,C*
035-21	T lymphoma	41 M	S	A haplo; MLC+	active disease	A-2,C,TBI-2
036-22	AA	30 M	U	HLA match; MLC+	N/A	C*,TBI-3
037-23	AML	14 F	F	A,B haplo; MLC+	M2A marrow-2nd remission	C,TBI-1

Fa = Father
S = Sister
B = Brother
U = Unrelated donor
N/A = Non Applicable
Mo = Mother
j = Juvenile type

N = Nitrogen mustard 1.5 mg/kg × 3 doses
B = Busulfan 4 mg/kg × 4 doses
A-1 = Cytosine arabinoside 200 mg/m^2 over 24 hrs × 2 doses
A-2 = Cytosine arabinoside 3 gms/m^2 × 6 doses over 72 hrs
C = Cyclophosphamide 60 mg/kg × 2 doses
C* = Cyclophosphamide 50 mg/kg × 4 doses
D = Daunomycin 40 mg/m^2 × 2 doses

TBI-1 = 1320 Rads given in 8 165 rad fx
TBI-2 = 1200 Rads given in 5 240 rad fx
TBI-3 = 300 Rads given in 2 150 rad fx
MLC+ = Reactive in mixed lymphocyte culture
MLC- = Nonreactive in mixed lymphocyte culture
WA = Wiskott Aldrich

of the antibody and complement treatment of the bone marrow to remove the T lymphocytes are described elsewhere.[27] The number of E-rosette positive cells and OKT3 positive cells found pre- and post treatment are detailed in Table 3. The dose of nucleated bone marrow cells remaining after treatment is also given in Table 3.

Assessment of Engraftment and GvHD

We defined the day of engraftment as the third consecutive day on which the white blood cell count was greater than 1,000 cells/mm^3 and increasing.[21] Whenever possible, we documented engraftment of the donor marrow with karyotypic analysis of bone marrow cells, HLA-phenotyping of peripheral blood lymphocytes, or red cell phenotyping. Two long-term survivors (020-06 and 024-10) had evidence of autologous recovery and are the subjects of a more extensive analysis of host-versus-graft immunity.

Table 2
Complement Dependent Cytotoxicity of CT-2

Cell Type Tested	No. Positive/No. Tested
Normal Cells	
T lymphocytes	102/102
B lymphocytes	0/9
Granulocytes	0/4
Monocytes	0/4
Platelets	0/2
Thymocytes	2/2
Leukemia Cells	
B CLL	0/7
T CLL	1/1
T ALL	5/5
Common ALL	0/7
AML	0/5
Cell Lines	
Daudi (B lymphoma)	negative
Conception (B lymphoma)	negative
Reh (Common ALL)	negative
IM9 (B line)	negative
HL60 (AML)	negative
8402 (T ALL)	negative
Molt 4 (T ALL)	20–30% positive
HPB ALL (T ALL)	80–100% positive
JM (T ALL)	10–20% positive
CEM (T ALL)	40–50% positive

Specificity testing of monoclonal antibody CT-2 was measured by cytotoxicity against panels of normal cells, leukemia cells, and cell lines. Measurement of positivity is a measure of percent of cells killed and detected by eosin dye exclusion assay.

We defined the severity of GvHD by the well-established Seattle criteria.[12] GvHD was initially treated with prednisone 1–2 mg/kg/day and if unresponsive, then the dose was increased to 500-1500 mg/day. Cyclosporine A, given in a dose of 5 mg/kg/day to patient 035-21 for well-established GvHD, resolved all signs of GvHD.

RESULTS

The clinical outcome of the 23 patients who received allogenic T lymphocyte-depleted bone marrow is shown in Tables 3, 4 and 5. All patients were followed up for at least 100 days post transplant or until death occurred.

HLA-Matched Recipients

Eight patients received fully matched allogenic bone marrow transplants. Seven of the eight were leukemic patients and engrafted promptly; patient 033-19 with AA had evidence of trilineage engraftment by 14 days after BMT, but rejected the graft over the ensuing seven days, necessitating a second transplant. Engraftment occurred 38 days after that second transplant. The mean time to engraftment in all eight patients following BMT was 23 days.

Only two of the eight fully matched patients developed GvHD; both were only of Grade 1 severity and both responded to low-dose prednisone. Except for patient 033-19 with aplastic anemia, who rejected the first bone marrow allograft and received prednisone and ATG after the second transplant to prevent rejection, none of the other seven patients received any GvHD prophylaxis. Five of the eight matched patients were older than 16 years. The mean dose of bone marrow given was 2.10×10^8 nucleated cells/kg as detailed in Table 4.

Two of the eight fully matched patients died from recurrent leukemia on days 181 and 219 post BMT. Four others died from infections. Two of these four developed evidence of immunoblastic lymphomas post BMT (016-02 and 033-19) and in one of these patients, the lymphoma was proved to be Epstein-Barr virus (EBV)-related.

HLA-Mismatched Recipients

Fifteen patients received allogenic histoincompatible bone marrow. The degree of identity is detailed in Table 1 and the clinical outcome of this group is shown in Table 5.

Two of the 15 patients, both with immunodeficiency, died prior to any signs of engraftment (034-20 and 037-23) from infection and pulmonary edema, respectively. One of these two patients failed to engraft

118

Table 3
Clinical Outcome for All 23 Patients Who Received T-Lymphocyte Depleted Marrow

UPN	BM Dose ($\times 10^8$ Nucleated Cells/kg)	Pre^{E+}	Post	Day of Engraft[2]	GvHD[3]	Outcome
012-01	3.17	24	0	16	0	relapsed day 199, died day 219
016-02	0.84	28.5	0	25	0	died day 180 pneumonia
017-03	5.80	23	0.2	27	0	relapsed day 48; died day 87
018-04	1.09	35.7	0.8	–	3	died day 43, infection
019-05	1.33	28	0	31	1	relapsed day 146, died day 181
020-06	0.99	20.4	0	–	0	
	1.68	34	0.6	–	0	alive >290 days
	3.21	46	0	–	0	
021-07	4.06	22.4	0.4	25	1	alive >280 days
022-08	2.44	30	0.1	48	4	died day 55, aspergillosis
	1.41	27	0			

Patient	Rosettes[1]		[2]	[3]		Outcome
023-09	8.08	32	0.1	—	0	died day 3, post BMT 2, cardiopulmonary edema
	8.36	23	0	—	1	alive, relapsed day 243
024-10	2.02	37	0.1	63	1	died day 111, fungus
025-11	2.01	38	0.5	—	0	
	2.94	37	0.1	—	0	alive >240 days
026-12	9.83	26	0.1	20	2	died day 14, infection
027-13	9.51	22	0	—	2	alive >230 days
028-14	11.31	22	0	32	0	alive >225 days
029-15	2.17	48	0	16	0	died day 80, CMV pneumonia
030-16	1.88	39	0.1	16	N/A	died day 24, infection
031-17	1.65	26	0.3	—	0	died day 38, hepatitis
032-18	2.54	27.5	0.2	14	0	died day 89, pneumonia, EBV infection
033-19	1.29	29.8	1.3	—	0	
	1.60	29.8	0	—	N/A	
034-20	4.99	8.1	0.1	—	4	died day 1, pneumonia
035-21	1.42	20	0.3	24	0	died day 53 due to pneumonia, recurrent tumor
036-22	2.64	25.6	0.1	—	0	died day 60, pneumonia
037-23	1.31	30.1	0.9	—	0	died day 55, pulmonary edema, infection

[1] Percent of cells pre- and post treatment that form rosettes with sheep red cells.
[2] Defined as the third consecutive day of a total WBC greater than 1000 cells/mm^3.
[3] Defined by Seattle criterion.

initially and was undergoing a second preparatory regimen for a second transplant. The other patient died one day after undergoing a BMT, and thus could not be evaluated for engraftment or GvHD.

Of the remaining 13 patients, only six showed evidence of engraftment as defined in this study. One additional patient (020-06) eventually reached a white count greater than 1000 cells/mm^3; however, this patient and one other who is a member of this group of 6/13 patients was documented to have only autologous recovery of bone marrow. These two patients, plus one other, will be described in more detail in another publication.

Only four of the original group of 15 survive at this time. Two of these four surviving patients had evidence of autologous recovery of cells. The other two (028-14 and 026-12) had immunodeficiency syndromes, and engraftment was documented by red cell-phenotyping and HLA-typing, or by the presence of donor T-cells when no T-cells had been evident prior to transplant.

Several of the mismatched patients who failed to engraft as defined in this study did have histologic evidence of early engraftment at the time of death. All three patients (017-03, 022-08 and 035-21) who received cytosine arabinoside in addition to the TBI and cyclophosphamide engrafted well. All three of these patients died. One child with juvenile CML died of recurrent leukemia and one other patient (022-08) died of disseminated aspergillosis. The third patient, transplanted at the time of lymphoma relapse (035-21), died of infection and recurrent tumor.

Because two of the 15 patients died before any bone marrow was evident, only 13 patients could be evaluated for occurrence of GvHD (Table 4). Ten of the 13 developed Grade 0-2 GvHD and only three of the 13

Table 4
BMT Summary Data, Matched Patients

Number of matched patients	8
Marrow dose (mean × 10^8 nucleated cells/kg)	2.10
Mean day of engraftment	23
Incidence of acute GvHD:	
Grade 0:	6/8
Grade 1:	2/8

Patient outcome:
  alive (2/8):   021-07 (>280 days); 029-15 (>225 days)

died:	#021-01:	relapsed on day 199, died day 219
	#016-02:	died day 180 pneumonia, fungus, lymphoma
	#019-05:	relapsed on day 146, died day 181
	#030-16:	died on day 80 CMV pneumonia
	#032-18:	died on day 38 viral hepatitis
	#033-19:	died on day 89 EBV infection, two fungal infections

developed Grade 3–4 GvHD. Of the six that engrafted, four developed GvHD (two with Grade 4 GvHD, one with Grade 2 GvHd and one with Grade 1 GvHD). No patient received methotrexate post transplant to prevent GvHD, although several received cyclophosphamide post transplant to prevent GvHD and/or graft rejection.

Recovery of T-lymphocyte subsets will be reported more completely elsewhere, but in all engrafted patients we documented T-lymphocyte recovery. Two of the mismatched patients who subsequently failed to engraft and died had evidence of an immunoblastic lymphoma present at autopsy, which may be related to an EBV infection.

There was a clear difference between the mismatched patients and the matched patients in regard to the occurrence of severe GvHD of Grade 2–4 (38% vs. 0%, respectively). All eight of the matched patients engrafted (although one patient with AA required retransplantation), whereas only six of the 15 mismatched patients engrafted, and one of these six, plus one additional surviving patient, eventually had only autologous cells detected in the bone marrow or peripheral blood.

Table 5
BMT Summary Data, Mismatched Patients

Number of mismatched patients	15
Marrow dose (mean $\times$ 10^8 nucleated cells/kg)	4.17
Mean day of engraftment*	38
Incidence of acute GvHD:†	
Grade 0:	6/13
Grade 1:	2/13
Grade 2:	2/13
Grade 3:	1/13
Grade 4:	2/13

Patient outcome:
alive (4/15): 020–06 (>290 days); 024–10 (>260 days)
               026–12 (>240 days); 028–14 (>230 days)

died: #017–03: relapsed on day 48, died on day 87
       #018–04: died on day 43, infection
       #022–08: died on day 55, aspergillosis
       #023–09: died on day 3, pulmonary edema and heart failure
       #025–11: died on day 111, fungus
       #027–13: died on day 14, infection
       #031–17: died on day 24, meningitis
       #034–20: died on day 1, pneumonia
       #035–21: died on day 53, pneumonia, recurrent tumor
       #036–22: died on day 60, pneumonia
       #037–23: died on day 55, pulmonary edema, fungus infections

*See text for definition of engraftment.
†2/15 of the patients died prior to engraftment and GvHD could not then be evaluated. Not included in the totals.

DISCUSSION

The results of the transplant experience on the first 23 patients reconstituted with T lymphocyte-depleted bone marrow indicate that the in vitro treatment of donor bone marrow is safe for both graft and recipient. All of those patients receiving matched, histocompatible bone marrow for leukemia (seven of seven) had evidence of prompt engraftment, and six of the 15 patients receiving histoincompatible bone marrow had evidence of engraftment, with one additional patient who only had autologous recovery.

All eight patients receiving fully matched HLA-MLC compatible bone marrow showed no evidence of severe GvHD (Grade 2–4). The only patient to receive any anti-GvHD prophylaxis was a child with AA who failed to engraft with her first transplant; she was retransplanted and received prednisone and ATG post transplant.

Five of 13 (38%) of our evaluable patients developed severe GvHD. In all cases the GvHD responded well to steroids or cyclosporine A. These results indicate that the incidence of GvHD for our patients was comparable to the reported rates for those receiving matched transplants with post-BMT methotrexate administered as anti-GvHD prophylaxis.

The occurrence of GvHD was, however, not the major problem in the mismatched patients. Delayed engraftment or failure of engraftment were the more common problems, and in two of the long-term survivors, only autologous recovery was documented. Both of these patients, and one additional patient who died before engrafting, gave evidence of autologous lymphocytes in the peripheral blood within the first few weeks post-BMT. This suggests that the ablative therapy for these patients did not sufficiently suppress the recipient's residual immune system to allow for the graft survival.

We infer from our experience, including the good engraftment in our three donor-mismatched patients who received more intensive immune ablation with cytosine arabinoside in addition to the cyclophosphamide and TBI, that all patients who receive histoincompatible bone marrow should receive more intensive ablation prior to transplant, and cyclosporine A post transplant[24] to prevent graft rejection. Early results on more recently engrafted patients who received T lymphocyte-depleted histoincompatible donor marrow suggest that, although the intensive immune ablation regimen is very toxic to heavily pretreated patients, engraftment is prompt and no different from graft outcome in patients who receive fully compatible transplants.

REFERENCES

1. Thomas ED, Buchner LD, Banaji M, et al: One hundred patients with acute leukemia treated by chemotherapy, total body irradiation and allogenic transplantation. *Blood* 1977;49:511.

2. Champlin R, Ho W, Winston DJ, et al: Allogenic bone marrow transplantation for chronic myelogenous leukemia in chronic or accelerated phase. *Transplant Proc* 1983;15:1401–1404.
3. Vowels MR, Lam-Po-Tang R, Heller E, et al: Bone marrow transplantation for acute leukemia in childhood. *Aust Paediatr J* 1982;18:264–276.
4. Thomas ED: Allogenic bone marrow transplantation for blood cell disorders. *Birth Defects* Original Article Series 1982;18:361–369.
5. Gale, RP: Bone marrow transplantation in leukemia. *Ann Clin Res* 1981;13:367–372.
6. Dupont B, Flomenberg N, OReilly RJ: Bone marrow transplantation for correction of severe aplastic anemia and primary immunodeficiency. *Ann Clin Res* 1981;13:358–366.
7. Johnson FL: Marrow transplantation in the treatment of acute childhood leukemia. *Ann J Pediatr Hem/Onc* 1981;3:389–395.
8. Beutler E, Blune KG, Bross KJ, et al: Bone marrow transplantation as the treatment of choice for "good risk" adult patients with leukemia. *Trans Assoc Am Physicians* 1979;42:189–195.
9. Storb R: Recent developments in allogenic marrow transplantation for the treatment of severe aplastic anemia. *Blut* 1981;43:339–344.
10. Buckner CD, Clift RA, Thomas ED, et al: Allogenic marrow transplantation for patients with acute non-lymphoblastic leukemia in second remission. *Leuk Res* 1982;6:395–399.
11. Buckner CD, Clift RA, Thomas ED: Bone marrow transplantation. *Leuk Res* 1982;6:381–382.
12. Thomas ED, Storb R, Clift RA, et al: Bone marrow transplantation. *N Engl J Med* 1975;292:832.
13. Tsoi MS, Storb R, Dobbs S, et al: Specific suppressor cells and immune response to host antigens in long-term human allogenic marrow recipients: Implications for the mechanisms of graft-versus-host tolerance and chronic graft-versus-host disease. *Transplant Proc*. In press.
14. Tutschika PJ, Bortin MM: Graft-versus-host disease. *Transplant Proc* 1981;13:1267.
15. Ramsay NKC, Kersey JH, Robinson LL, et al: A randomized study of the prevention of acute graft-versus-host disease. *N Engl J Med* 1982;306:392.
16. Haas RJ, Janka G, Netzel B, et al: Antibody incubation of human marrow graft for prevention of graft-versus-host disease. *Blut* 1980;40:387.
17. Rodt H, Kolb HJ, Netzel B, et al: Effect of anti-T-cell globulin on GvHD in leukemia patients treated with BMT. *Transplant Proc* 1981;13:257.
18. Granger S, Janossy G, Francis G, et al: Elimination of T lymphocytes from human bone marrow with monoclonal T-antibodies and cytolytic complement. *Br J Haematol* 1982;50:367.
19. Reinherz EL, Geha R, Rappeport JM, et al: Reconstitution after transplantation with T lymphocyte depleted HLA haplotype-mismatched bone marrow for severe combined immunodeficiency. *Proc Natl Acad Sci USA* 1982;79:6047–6051.
20. Prentice HG, Janossy G, Skeggs D, et al: Use of anti-T-cell monoclonal antibody OKT3 to prevent acute graft-versus-host disease in allogenic bone marrow transplantation for acute leukemia. *Lancet* 1982;1:700.
21. Filipovich AH, Ramsay NKC, Warkentin PI, et al: Pretreatment of donor bone marrow with monoclonal antibody OKT3 for prevention of acute graft-versus-host disease in allogenic histocompatible bone marrow transplantation. *Lancet* 1982;1:1266.
22. Reisner Y, Kapoor N, Kirkpatrick D, et al: Transplantation for severe com-

bined immunodeficiency with HLA-A B, D, DR incompatible parental marrow cells fractionated by soybean agglutinin and sheep red blood cells. *Blood* 1983;61:341–348.

23. O'Reilly RJ, Kapoor N, Kirkpatrick D, et al: Transplantation for severe combined immunodeficiency using histoincompatible parental marrow fractionated by soybean agglutinin and sheep red blood cells: experience in six consecutive cases. *Transplant Proc* 1983;15:1431–1436.

24. Biggs JC, Atkinson K, Hayes J, et al: After allogenic bone marrow transplantation, Cyclosprine A is associated with faster engraftment, less mucositis, and three distinct syndromes of nephrotoxicity when compared to methotrexate. *Transplant Proc* 1983;15:1487–1489.

25. Thierfelder S, Hoffmann-Fezer G, Rodt H, et al: Antilymphocytic antibodies and marrow transplantation. *Transplantation* 1983;35:249–254.

26. Vallera DA, Soderling CCB, Carlson GJ, et al: Bone marrow transplantation across major histocompatibility barriers in mice. *Transplantation* 1981;31:218.

27. Trigg ME, Billing R, Sondel PM, et al: In vitro treatment of donor bone marrow with anti-E-rosette antibody and complement prior to transplantation. *J Cell Biochem* 1983;7A:57.

Use of Monoclonal Antibodies and Rabbit Serum Complement for 2–3 Log Depletion of T Cells in Donor Marrow

P.J. Marin, J.A. Hansen, E.D. Thomas

We have initiated a clinical pilot trial to evaluate the use of murine monoclonal anti-T cell antibodies and rabbit serum complement to remove T cells from donor marrow as a means of preventing graft-versus-host disease (GvHD) after HLA-matched allogenic marrow transplantation. In our protocol, donor-marrow mononuclear cells are first prepared by centrifugation on Ficoll-Hypaque (S.G. 1.077) gradients. The cells are incubated for 30 minutes at 4C with a mixture of eight different anti-T cell antibodies, each at saturating concentrations. The antibodies were purified from ascites fluid by affinity chromatography on Protein A-sepharose columns. Washed cells are then incubated twice with 50 ml of selected rabbit serum complement for 60 minutes at 37C. T cells in the pretreatment marrow are enumerated by indirect immunofluorescence and flow microfluorimetry. The patients are treated with cyclosporine for prophylaxis of GHD. The following table details representative results for two patients:

Patient	Original Number T cells ($\times 10^9$)	Cells Infused (per kg)			Engraftment Day	
		Nucleated ($\times 10^6$)	BFU-E ($\times 10^3$)	CFU-C ($\times 10^3$)	WBC ≥ 100	WBC ≥ 500
1	1.63	54	37	52	9	11
2	1.36	85	22	33	11	15

Samples of treated marrow cells were cultured for 7 days in medium containing 1 μg/ml PHA, and then stained by indirect immunofluorescence with a mixture of anti-T cells antibodies. T-cell blasts were not detected in these cultured cells, indicating that the frequency of T cells remaining and administered to the patient was less than 1/2000. Our results demonstrate the feasibility of using monoclonal antibodies and modest amounts of rabbit serum (100 cc) to achieve 2–3 logs of T-cell lysis without apparent damage to stem cells necessary for engraftment. Evaluation of the effectiveness of this procedure for prevention of GvHD will require a larger number of patients and further follow-up.

14 Phase I Study of High-Dose Serotherapy with Cytotoxic Monoclonal Antibodies in Patients with Gastrointestinal Malignancies

S.I. Drew, P.I. Terasaki, C. Johnson,
D. Chia, A. Wakisaka, S. Hardiwidjaja,
J. Cicciarelli, M. Takasugi,
P. Kaszubowski, T. Quinlan,
T. Izuka, A. Hirata

Utilizing the hybridoma technology[1] to develop monoclonal antibodies to antigens present on certain gastrointestinal cancer cells, we initiated a phase 1 study of patients with esophageal, pancreatic, colon, and gastric adenocarcinomas. Our approach differed from previous serotherapy trials in that the antibodies utilized were (a) cytotoxic in vitro with human complement; (b) administered in large doses in rapidly escalating dose schedules; and (c) given in conjunction with fresh frozen plasma and, in certain cases, lymphocyte-enriched preparations so as to augment the endogenous humoral and cell-mediated immune responses. This report deals with the first three of eight patients treated with monoclonal antibodies CES01 and CCOL1.

METHODS AND MATERIALS

Patients

Consenting adult patients with gastrointestinal tumors were treated as part of a phase 1 study of monoclonal antibody serotherapy. The clinical features of the patients are shown in Table 1. All patients had locally invasive or metastatic tumors that had failed conventional surgery, chemotherapy, and radiation therapy.

Monoclonal Antibodies

Two monoclonal antibodies, CES01 and CCOL1,[2] utilized for serotherapy, react specifically against esophageal squamous cell carcinoma

Table 1
Clinical Features of Patients Receiving Monoclonal Antibody Therapy

Patient	Tumor Type	Previous Therapy†	Estimated Tumor Mass (g)‡	Skin Test	Toxicity§	Serum Sickness	Clinical Course
1	esophagus*	S, R	<20	3 cm erythema	Nil	–	Death from aspiration Tumor present at autopsy
2 (course 1) (course 2)	colon	S, C	>100	negative erythema	Nil Nil	– –	Rising CEA, progressive disease → death
3	pancreas	C	>100	negative	V, D	+	Rising CEA, progressive disease → death

*Squamous cell carcinoma; all other tumors adenocarcinomas.
†S: surgery; R: radiation therapy; C: chemotherapy.
‡Sum of the volume of individual tumor masses ($\Sigma\ 4/3\ \Pi r^3$).
§V: vomiting; D: diarrhea.

(CES01) and stomach, colonic, and pancreatic adenocarcinomas (CCOL1), respectively. Testing by immunoperoxidase, cytotoxicity, and the ELISA assay showed no significant reactivity of the antibodies against a panel of normal tissues and peripheral blood cells. An ammonium sulfate precipitate of both antibodies was prepared in accordance with all of the biologic criteria required by the Food and Drug Administration for use of these reagents in human trials. In particular, the antibodies were found to be sterile and free of endotoxins and murine viruses. Purification of the antibodies into immunoglobulin fractions for in vivo use was not performed. Measurement of specific immunoglobulin levels in all antibody lots utilized showed that the IgG fraction comprised greater than 50% of the mouse ascites infusate. Both antibodies are cytotoxic for their respective target cells in the presence of human complement.

Administration of Monoclonal Antibodies

Testing of pretreatment biopsy specimens showed that the antibodies reacted positively (over 75% of the malignant cells stained or killed in vitro) to the tumor tissue. Following preliminary skin testing, the antibodies were infused in 100–200 ml of normal saline through a peripheral vein over 60 to 90 minutes. Pre- and post treatment sera samples were drawn for biological studies. Evidence of toxicity as well as therapeutic responses were monitored by clinical evaluation and routine biochemical and radiographic studies. Monoclonal antibodies were given in rapidly incremental doses as outlined in Table 2. In all patients, two antibody doses were administered on day 1 of therapy to exclude acute allergic reactions before initiating the escalating dose schedule. Patients 2 and 3 received fresh frozen plasma with doses of antibody of 500 mg (see Table 2). In addition, infusions of lymphocyte-enriched preparations were administered to patient 2 during his second course of therapy.

Biological Assays

Antibody titers in human serum were measured by a standard microcytotoxicity assay[3] using the target cell lines SH (esophageal carcinoma cell line) or 205 (colon cancer cell line) and human complement as a lytic source. Staining of the tissue specimens was performed by immunoperoxidase[4] or immunofluorescence.[5] The enzyme-linked immunoassay (ELISA)[2] was used to semiquantitate serum levels of mouse immunoglobulin and human antimurine antibodies (HAMA). Total hemolytic complement, C3, and C4 levels were measured by radioimmunodiffusion (Kallestad Quantiplate, MN). Antibody-dependent cellular cytotoxicity using monoclonal antibody-coated target cells and normal effector lymphocytes was performed as previously described.[6]

130

Table 2
Dose Schedule of Monoclonal Antibody Serotherapy

Day	1 Mon	2 Tues	3 Wed	4 Thurs	5 Fri	7	9	11	13	Total Dose (mg)
Patient 1	1, 10	40	110	318						479
2 (course 1)	2, 20	150	350	600	1000	500*†				2122
2 (course 2)	1,10	100	500*†	500*†	*		500*†	500*	500*†	3111
3	1,10	100	500*				100*	100*	200*	1011

Two doses of antibody are administered on day 1.
*Two units of fresh frozen plasma.
†Packed lymphocyte infusion.

RESULTS

Clinical Outcome and Toxicity

Patients 1 and 2 demonstrated a positive erythema reaction to the pretreatment intradermal skin test. None of these patients went on to develop evidence of acute allergic reactions. Furthermore, the occurrence of serum sickness (see below) did not appear to correlate with the skin test outcome. In patient 3, following the 500 mg antibody dose, vomiting and diarrhea on day 3 occurred, necessitating intravenous fluid resuscitation for about one week. No evidence of acute allergic reaction, gastrointestinal bleeding, or alteration in hematologic values, serum amylase levels, or liver and kidney function tests was noted during any course of antibody therapy. Evidence of serum sickness, including a rash, fever, chills, and arthralgia, developed in patient 3 approximately four hours following antibody administration on days 9, 11, and 13. Symptoms persisted for approximately 24 hours. Because of the allergic reactions, antibody therapy was discontinued. All evidence of serum sickness resolved spontaneously without the use of corticosteroids.

By clinical, radiographic or tumor marker (CEA) criteria, no evidence of tumor regression was noted in any of the patients treated with monoclonal antibody therapy. All three patients subsequently died two to six months following completion of therapy. Rising CEA titers were noted in patients 2 and 3. In patient 1, death occurred as a result of food aspiration, and the autopsy revealed the presence of a 2-cm retrocardiac tumor deposit. Permission for autopsy was not granted in the other two patients.

Immunopathological studies (ie, in vivo localization of antibody) were undertaken in patient 2 following the administration of antibody on day 5 (course 1). Positive cellular staining with the CCOL1 antibody by direct immunoperoxidase was noted in the biopsy of a tumor-bearing supraclavicular lymph node. Staining of tumor tissue was focal in distribution and did not involve the entire metastatic deposit in the node.

Serum Monoclonal Antibody Titers

Serum titers of antibody were measured at intervals following the administration of each dose. Following doses of 500 mg or more, measurable titers of the CCOL1 antibody were detected for at least 48 hours. The profiles of the antibody titers are shown in Figures 1, 2, 3, and Table 3.

Mouse Immunoglobulin Levels

Serum levels of mouse immunoglobulin were measured (Figures 1, 2 and 3) and shown to remain elevated for periods longer than the

132

measurable titer of specific antibody. Based on data obtained from other patients (unpublished), levels of mouse immunoglobulin return to baseline usually with seven days following completion of antibody therapy. The variation noted in the clearance between mouse immunoglobulin and specific antibody possibly reflects fixation of specific antibody by the target antigens, development of an anti-idiotype response to the monoclonal antibody or differences in the clearance of individual components of the mouse ascites infusate.

Table 3
Patient #1—Serum Antibody Titer*

	Day 1	2	3	4
Antibody (mg)	*11*	*40*	*110*	*318*
Pre-treatment	0	0	0	0
Post treatment				
0 min	8	64	128	128
15 min	2	64	64	256
45 min	0	32	64	256
105 min	0	8	32	256
24 hours	0	0	0	0

*Reciprocal titer.

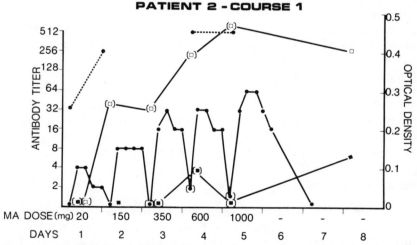

Figure 1 Progressive increments in the cytotoxic titer of monoclonal antibody (MA) CCOL1 during the initial infusion of large daily doses of antibody (solid circles joined by a solid line). In patient 2, serum levels of human antimouse antibodies (HAMA, solid squares joined by a solid line) and mouse immunoglobulin (open squares joined by a solid line) are shown (ELISA assay, optical density). Parentheses indicate preinfusion titers. MA titer in intravenous tubing shown by solid circles joined by a broken line.

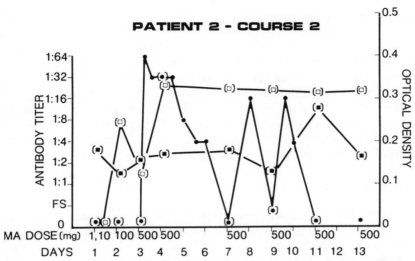

Figure 2 Monoclonal antibody titers (solid circles joing by a solid line) in the serum of patient 2 during the second serotherapy course. Levels of HAMA (solid squares joined by a solid line) are elevated as a result of immunization following course 1 therapy. Note measurable serum titers of MA in presence of HAMA following infusion of large (500 mg) doses of antibody.

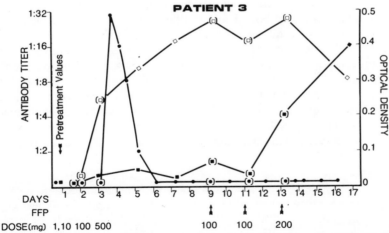

Figure 3 Monoclonal antibody titers in serum of patient 3 (solid circles joined by solid line). Immunization with MA evident by rise in HAMA levels (solid squares joined by solid line).

Human Antimurine Antibodies

Immunization of patients with mouse immunoglobulin was monitored during the serotherapy courses. In patient 1, no HAMA response was observed up to one month following therapy. Conversely, patients 2 and 3 developed an antimurine response (Figures 2 and 3), and in the latter patient, this was associated with clinical evidence of serum sickness. In patient 2 (course 2), antibody doses of 500 mg administered in the presence of HAMA produced no untoward clinical reactions, and also resulted in measurable titers of specific antibody.

Serum Complement Levels

Total hemolytic complement, C3 and C4 were measured in each patient during the serotherapy course. The reduction in the total hemolytic complement and C4 levels was noted in all of the patients and, in particular, in patient 2. The depletion of complement following the injection of antibody suggested the fixation of complement in vivo. Efforts to boost complement levels by infusion of fresh frozen plasma failed to increase the serum C4 values, and could be responsible in part for the limited efficacy of the antibody serotherapy. Full details of the complement fluctuation is given in a separate report in this issue.

Cell-Mediated Immunity

Serum from patient 3 was studied for its effect on autologous antibody-dependent cellular cytotoxicity (ADCC) using third-party normal effector lymphocytes and cultured tumor cells (ST) established from a sample of peritoneal lavage fluid obtained from the same patient. Cultured cells were coated with the patient's serum and incubated with effector lymphocytes. Although tumor cell lysis was present during the initial days of serotherapy, blocking of ADCC was noted by day 9 of therapy and corresponded with the development of HAMA in the patient's serum. The same serum inhibited an independent ADCC assay comprising normal effector cells and antilymphocyte-serum-coated lymphocytes (data not shown), demonstrating the nonspecificity of the reaction.

DISCUSSION

The therapeutic potential of passively administered monoclonal antibodies in patients with lymphoma,[7] leukemia[7] and gastrointestinal tumors[8] is currently under study. Despite the curative outcome in one patient with end-stage lymphoma,[9] no definite responses have been noted in solid tumors of the gastrointestinal tract. Of the four patients with metastatic gastrointestinal tumors treated by Sears et al,[8] a minor response was noted in one patient.

Using antibodies that are cytotoxic in vitro with human complement, we attempted to treat three patients with metastatic gastrointestinal tumors, employing high doses of antibody in a rapidly escalating dose schedule. The schedule was selected purposely to ensure that adequate doses were administered before the onset of human antimurine responses by the host. Overall, no significant clinical or biochemical evidence of toxicity was observed. Only in patient 3 was there evidence of nausea and vomiting that required intravenous fluid replenishment following administration of 500 mg of antibody. There was no correlation between skin test results and the development of subsequent acute or delayed allergic reactions. The delayed allergic reactions in patient 3 could be attributed to the presence of human antimurine antibodies, and was exacerbated by administration of the monoclonal antibody. Conversely, even in the presence of human antimurine antibodies in patient 2 (course 2), no acute allergic reactions or serum sickness were noted despite the continued administration of antibody. The reasons for the difference in clinical reactions in the two patients is unclear.

In all three patients, no objective evidence of tumor response was noted despite evidence suggesting that in vivo binding of the antibody to the tumor tissue does occur. Binding of antibody to tumor cells in vivo has been confirmed in other patients 24 hours following antibody administration (unpublished). Whereas primary tumors often stain homogeneously with antibody, focal staining of biopsy specimens of metastatic sites is more common and highlights the likely clonal heterogeneity of solid tumors.[10]

Failure to observe a therapeutic response in the treated patients is certainly multifactoral and may be related to: (a) an excessive tumor burden in patients 2 and 3; (b) tumor heterogeneity; (c) complement consumption despite supplementation with fresh frozen plasma (Figures 2, 3); and (d) blockage of endogenous cell-mediated immunity by monoclonal antibody-human antimurine antibody-immune complexes (Figure 4). Based on these suppositions, future direction in monoclonal-antibody serotherapy should therefore address the following issues: (a) treatment of patients with limited tumor burdens; (b) the possible use of combination antibody therapy to overcome tumor heterogeneity; (c) vigorous attempts at in vivo complement supplementation when using complement-binding antibodies; (d) induction of host tolerance to murine antibodies or the use of human monoclonal antibodies; and (e) utilization of antibody in conjunction with radionuclides, toxins, chemotherapy agents and possibly hyperthermia. Our preliminary observations showing blocking of in vivo cellular immunity[11] should caution investigators as to the possibility that antibody serotherapy may possibly enhance tumor growth.

136

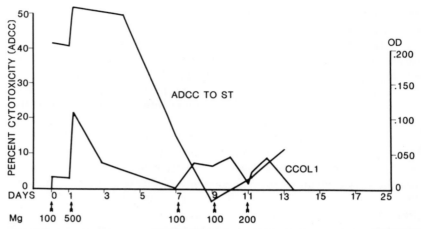

Figure 4 Serotherapy in patient 3 showing disappearance of specific ADCC to autologous cultured tumor cells (ST) by day 9 and the serum levels of CCOL1.

REFERENCES

1. Kohler B, Millstein C: Continuous cultures of fused cells secreting antibody of predefined specificity. *Nature* 1975;256:495–497.
2. Kaszubowski PA, Terasaki PI, Chia DS, et al: A cytotoxic monoclonal antibody to clonal adenocarcinoma. *Cancer Res* (in press).
3. Terasaki PI, Bernoco D, Park MS, et al: Microdroplet testing for HLA-A, -B, -C and -D antigens. *Am J Clin Pathol* 1978;69:103–120.
4. Colcher D, Hand PH, Teramoto YA, et al: Use of monoclonal antibodies to define the diversity of mammary tumor viral gene products in virions and mammary tumors of the genus mus. *Cancer Res* 1981;41:1451–1459.
5. Galton J, Ivanyi J: An immunofluorescent technique for the detection of lymphocyte alloantigens. *J Immunol Methods* 1977;17:57–61.
6. Takasugi M, Mickey MR, Levine PH. Natural and antibody-dependent cell-mediated cytotoxicity to cultured target cells superinfected with Epstein-Barr virus. *Cancer Res* 1982;43:1208–1214.
7. Ritz J, Schlossman SF: Utilization of monoclonal antibodies in the treatment of leukemia and lymphoma. *Blood* 1982;59:1–11.
8. Sears HF, Mattis J, Herlyn D, et al: Phase 1 clinical trial of monoclonal antibody in treatment of gastrointestinal tumors. *Lancet* 1982;1:762–765.
9. Miller RA, Malone DG, Warnke MD, et al: Treatment of B-cell lymphoma with monoclonal anti-idiotype antibody. *N Engl J Med* 1982;306:517.
10. Tumor cell heterogeneity, in Owens A, Coffey D, Baylin S (eds): *Bristol Meyers Symposium on Cancer Research*, vol 4, 1982.
11. Takasugi M, Drew SI, Kaszubowski P, et al: Disappearnce of specific autologous antibody-dependent cell-mediated cytotoxicity to a tumor following monoclonal antibody immunotherapy (submitted).

15 Complement Levels in Cancer Patients Treated with Monoclonal Antibodies

J. Cicciarelli, P.I. Terasaki, K. Tokita,
S.I. Drew, S. Lemkin, G. Sherman,
T. Quinlan, C. Johnson, L. Blyn,
D. Chia, P. Kaszubowski

The UCLA Tissue Typing Laboratory has attempted to develop monoclonal antibodies (MCA) for treatment of human solid tumors and leukemias and also for the amelioration of graft rejection episodes in human kidney transplantation. Large-scale cytotoxicity screening procedures have enabled us to find these complement-fixing MCA from hybridoma cells.

The reasons for selection of complement-fixing antibodies, and specifically, antibodies that use human serum as a complement source, has been two-fold. First, complement-fixing antibodies, as determined by the microtoxicity test,[1] may be a good in vitro correlate for the ability of the antibody to kill tumor cells in vivo. Second, not only does complement produce lysis of the target cell by activation of complement components 8 and 9, but other complement components produce opsoninization and chemotaxis, that is, the marshaling of cellular elements to the tumor cell antigen and the destruction and elimination of the antigen.[2,3]

CCOL1, a MCA that we found, is noncytotoxic with a panel of normal cells, but cytotoxic with complement to two colon adenocarcinoma cell lines, and by immunoperoxidase testing, to nine of 12 colon cancers and four of five pancreas cancers.[4] This antibody is highly specific to tumor cells and has limited amount of cross-reactivity to normal cells. It reacts to the atypical portions of the columnar epithelium in the intestine, albeit weakly. We therefore believed that this might be an appropriate antibody for serotherapy in solid tumors of the colon and pancreas.

The first patients treated with this antibody had large amounts of tumor (ie, > 50 g). Therefore, we decided to use as much antibody as was available to reduce tumor mass. Because of the large tumor amounts and the large amounts of antibody used, the patients' sera were examined for total hemolytic complement activity.

In this study, we will show that the complement levels decreased markedly (in some cases to zero) in patients with advanced disease, and that these changes in complement levels were a direct consequence of the infusion of large amount of CCOL1 antibody.

MATERIALS AND METHODS

Patients were part of a phase I/II clinical trial that determined both the toxicity and efficacy of CCOL1. Two patients with greater than 50 grams of tumor were treated at UCLA. The first was a colorectal adenocarcinoma patient and the second had pancreatic adenocarcinoma. The patients were treated with CCOL1 antibody according to a regimen outlined by Drew et al elsewhere in this book. Patients from Torrance Memorial Hospital were entered into the treatment protocol on the basis of less than 50 g of primary and metastatic disease and strong positive reactivity of the tumor to CCOL1. Complement levels were determined on quantaplates (Kallestad Laboratories, Austin, TX). All complement samples were determined on blood samples which were clotted and the sera were frozen immediately at −70C until testing.

RESULTS

The first UCLA patient was treated in the first course with approximately 2122 mg of an antibody that was ammonium sulfate-purified from mouse ascites. The doses were graduated from low to high and administered over a five day course so that primary antibody response would not have a chance to occur. The total hemolytic complement levels decreased gradually in response to the MCA (Figure 1). Total hemolytic complement levels dropped to zero (ie, nondetectable amounts) after 600 mg antibody infusion, subsequently rebounding after a 24-hour period. On day 5, when 1000 mg of antibody was infused, complement levels decreased to zero (nondetectable amounts) and stayed at that level for a 24-hour period. Figure 1 also shows that the complement component C4 was the limiting component. That is, C4 correlated exactly with the total hemolytic complement levels decreasing to zero. Further, C4 decreased in association with the infusion of the antibody.

Because of this correlation between the amount of infused antibody and the patient's complement level, all subsequent patients were transfused with frozen or fresh plasma as an exogenous complement source when the higher amounts of antibody were infused.

The second UCLA patient with advanced pancreatic cancer was given fresh frozen plasma with higher doses of antibody. However, therapy had to be discontinued after 500 mg infusion because of an adverse reaction (Drew et al, this volume). Because of low complement levels associated with infusion of CCOL1 we judged that these patients were not a good test to determine efficacious activity.

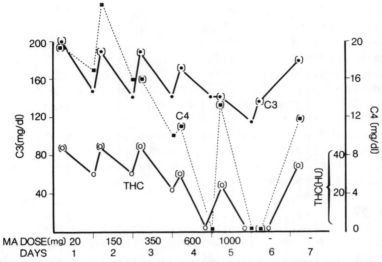

Figure 1 THC = total hemolytic complement; C4 = complement component 4; C3 = complement component 3.

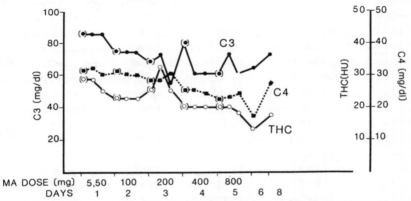

Figure 2 THC = total hemolytic complement; C4 = complement component 4; C3 = complement component 3.

Subsequent patients were chosen at Torrance Memorial Hospital in Torrance, CA, on the basis of a positive reaction of their tumor cells with MCA and tumor load of less than 50 grams as judged by a CAT scan. The first patients at Torrance Memorial Hospital were given 1500 mg of antibody. Figure 2 shows the treatment of one patient with colorectal cancer and the subsequent assay for his complement levels after antibody infusion. There is very little decrease in total hemolytic complement associated with the infusion of the monoclonal antibody in this patient (Figure 2). However, these patients received fresh frozen complement in the form of plasma at the time of 400 and 800 mg antibody infusion.

140

Figure 3 shows complement levels of another patient treated at Torrance Memorial Hospital that showed a decrease. However, the decrease was not to zero or undetectable levels, and so complement was still available for fixation onto antibodies that reacted to the appropriate tumor antigens. But a clear decrease in the total hemolytic complement was apparent upon the injection of 400 and 800 mg quantities of the antibody (Figure 3), indicating complement utilization associated with CCOL1 infusion.

Although it is too early to determine the clinical efficacy of the MCA serotherapy, we have observed no objective decrease in the amount of tumor even in those subjects in whom complement levels in the serum were maintained in physiological amounts.

DISCUSSION

In cancer patients with advanced disease and treated with a large amount of infused MCA, we were not surprised to see decreased complement levels. However, we were surprised that the complement levels dropped to zero or undetectable levels. This undetectable complement level seems to be associated with a decrease in complement component 4, and this was the rate-limiting component in the complement cascade. In these patients, there was a lack of objective tumor regression and both patients died. However, this may have occurred because the patients had advanced disease and the complement-fixing antibody did not have enough complement to effectively kill the tumor.

Because of these considerations, in subsequent experiments on the infusion of monoclonal antibody for therapy, we tested only those patients with a 50 g or less tumor burden. In five patients treated with MCA

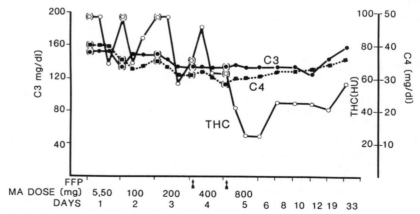

Figure 3 THC = total hemolytic complement; C4 = complement component 4; C3 = complement component 3.

who had 50 g or less of tumor, we were again unable to see objective criteria for the reduction of the tumor.

Initially, we believed that the lack of objective tumor regression was because of the reduced complement level associated with the infusion of CCOL1 antibody. However, after examining additional patients with smaller amounts of tumor and physiologically maintained complement levels, we believe that the lack of objective tumor regression in these patients may indeed mean that there are other mechanisms by which the tumors are escaping destruction by the MCA.

CCOL1 has tumor-killing ability in vitro by microtoxicity testing, and in vivo by mouse experiments in which the antibody binds and partially kills human tumors growing in nude mice (Table 1). In the paper by Drew et al, CCOL1 reacted in antibody-dependent cellular cytotoxicity. We also know that this antibody reacts to normal intestinal mucosa. The possible reasons for the antibody showing no effectiveness against tumors in patients with 50 g or less of tumor is outlined in Table 1.

First, the tumor mass and vascularity may be such that when the antibody is injected intravenously, even though CCOL1 binds to the tumor, it does not penetrate because it has to penetrate several layers of tissue before it gets to all of the tumor. Further, the tumor mass itself, and/or necrotic anaerobic areas of the tumor, may disallow the effective chemotaxis of blood elements and even complement components, so that the tumor is not killed. Although we have seen no evidence for antigenic modulation[5] with the particular antigen that CCOL1 recognizes, this is still a possibility and must be looked at with regard to antibodies used for serotherapy.

When one considers the kinetics of tumor growth, it may be that we are unable to detect a significant killing of tumor cells because the tumor itself is growing so quickly, and that even though the tumor is being destroyed, it appears not to change in size. Indeed, when we first detected the drop in complement associated with antibody infusion in the initial

Table 1

I.   Action of complement-fixing antibody (CCOL1)
- A. Tumor killing in vitro, in vivo (nude mice)
- B. Antibody-dependent cellular cytotoxicity (ADCC)
- C. Reactivity to normal mucosa

II.   Possible reasons for the tumor not showing a reduction in mass
- A. Tumor mass and vascularity
- B. Tumor antigen modulation
- C. Tumor growth kinetics
- D. Tumor growth enhancement (immunosuppression)
- E. Tumor heterogeneity
- F. Tumor antigen blocking
- G. Human antimurine antibody

142

patients who were treated without fresh frozen plasma, we though it indicated that the antibody was destroying the tumor even though we could not see any kind of definitive change in size. Further, in the nude mouse with growing human tumor there is a partial killing of the tumor, as shown by histologic sections, but there is no gross visible decrease in tumor size.

The possible enhancement of tumor growth by the injection of MCA must be considered. Tumor growth may be enhanced by the interdiction of some immune mechanism, as shown by Takasugi et al.[6] Tumor heterogeneity may play an important role in the effectiveness of treatment with MCA. Antigens that are recognized by some have been found on only part of the cancer cells.[7] Indeed, we found heterogeneity with regard to the antigen recognized by CCOL1. Because of heterogeneity of the tumor, we feel that MCA will be used in "cocktails" of MCA recognizing different tumor-associated antigens.

Antigens that are shed and/or secreted by the tumor and react to the MCA can block the binding of the antibody at the tumor site. However, this does not occur with CCOL1.

Finally, a problem that is universal in murine therapy is the production by the patient of human antimurine antibody (HAMA). When one treats a patient with murine monoclonals, there is a seven-day window in which to treat; after that time we have found HAMA in all of the patients treated to date with CCOL1. Until we are able to specifically suppress the HAMA response, there is only one time period in which to treat the patient.

Even though MCA has shown a limited efficacy in therapy of cancer patients,[8] there is enormous potential for treatment and cure of these patients.

REFERENCES

1. Cicciarelli J, Foon K, Terasaki P: Leukocyte antigens, in Cline M (ed): *Methods in Hematology*. London, Churchill Livingstone, 1981, p 84.
2. Muller-Eberhard H: Complement abnormalities in human disease. *Hosp Pract* 1978;12:65.
3. Colter H, Alper C, Rosen F: Genetics and biosynthesis of complement proteins. *N Engl J Med* 1981;304:653.
4. Kaszubowski PA, Terasaki PI, Chia DS, et al: A cytotoxic monoclonal antibody to colon adenocarcinoma. *Cancer Res* (in press).
5. Ritz J, Schlossman SF: Utilization of monoclonal antibodies in the treatment of leukemia and lymphoma. *Blood* 1982;59:1–11.
6. Takasugi M, Drew SI, Kaszubowski P, et al: Disappearance of specific autologous antibody-dependent cell-mediated cytotoxicity to a tumor following monoclonal antibody immunotherapy (submitted).
7. Owens A, Coffey D, Baylin S (eds): Tumor cell heterogeneity. *Bristol Meyers Symposium on Cancer Research*, vol 4, 1982.
8. Miner RA, Maloney DG, Warnice MD, et al: Treatment of B-cell lymphoma with monoclonal anti-idiotype antibody. *N Engl J Med* 1982;306:517.

16 Radioimmunoimaging in Malignant Melanoma Using ^{111}Indium-Labeled Anti-P-97 Monoclonal Antibody

J.L. Murray, E.M. Hersh,
M. Rosenblum, T.P. Haynie,
H. Glenn, J.M. Reuben, M.F. Hahns,
R.S. Benjamin, B.S. Yap,
C. Plager, N. Papadopoulos,
J. Frincke, D.L. Carlo

In 1948, Pressmann and Keighley showed that antisera produced against rat kidney could be successfully iodinated without loss of specificity. Subsequently, considerable work has been done using radiolabeled polyclonal antibodies to detect human tumors implanted in nude mice and in patients with solid tumors.[1,2] These studies were often difficult to perform because polyclonal antibodies to tumors were of low titer, low affinity, and contained variable amounts of contaminating proteins. Impure preparations were responsible for high background activity that detracted from actual uptake by tumor. Hence, the advent of high-titer, high-affinity monoclonal antibodies, specific for tumor-associated antigens, has rekindled interest in the area of radioimmunoimaging. Recently, a series of mouse monoclonal antibodies have been generated against several different epitopes of tumor-associated antigens found on a melanoma cell line.[3] One of these antibodies, designated P-96.5, reacted with over 80% of human melanoma cell lines and fresh tumor tissues.[4] This antibody has been successfully coupled to indium 111 and is available for imaging studies (Hybritech Inc). We present the preliminary results of a Phase I radioimmunoimaging study in malignant melanoma patients using this preparation.

SUBJECTS AND METHODS

Preparation of ^{111}In-Labeled P-96.5 Antibody

The P-97 antigen is a 97,000 dalton protein found on over 80% of melanoma cell lines and cell extracts. The antibody was derived from ascites

143

fluid of BALB/C mice using hybridoma technology as described previously.[5] The antibody was made by fusing BALB/C mouse spleen cells, immunized with a melanoma cell line, SK-Mel 28, with the NS-1 mouse myeloma cell line and selecting on Staphlococcus Aureus protein A coupled to sepharose CL-4B (Pharmacia). P-96.5 is of the IgG 2A subclass, is cytotoxic to melanoma cell lines in the presence of rabbit complement, and can mediate antibody-dependent cellular cytotoxicity.[6] It was provided by Hybritech is vials already bound to the bifunctional chelating agent (DTPA) and was ready for use following the addition of ^{111}In.

Patients

Twenty-one patients with malignant melanoma were studied. Only nonpregnant adults with stage III-B or IV-B metastic malignant melanoma (M.D. Anderson classification), as documented by appropriate x-rays and radionucleide scans, were eligible. There were 14 males and 7 females, with a median age of 42 years. One patient had a single axillary lymph node metastasis regional to the primary site and was classified as stage III-B. The remaining 20 patients had distant metastatic disease and were classified as stage IVB. Over one-half of the patients had received previous radiation therapy and/or chemotherapy prior to study. One patient was excluded because of a positive skin test (see below). In the remaining 20, there was a total of 41 metastatic tumor sites previously identified by x-rays, computed axial tomography, and radionucleide scans. The most frequent sites of involvement were lymph nodes in ten patients, lung in eight, and skin in six. Six of these 20 patients had a solitary metastatic site, whereas the remaining patients had multiple areas of metastases. Patients were not on therapy on the day of injection.

Study Plan

Following an initial history and physical examination, chest x-ray, EKG, CBC, platelet count, SMA-1260, and urinalysis, patients were skin tested with 0.1 μg P-96.5 monoclonal antibody. Skin tests were examined at one hour and 24 hours. Prior to study, blood was also drawn for in vitro immunologic tests. Whenever possible, patients with accessible tumor had biopsies performed for in vitro testing with the monoclonal antibody. All patients received a total of 2.5 mCi of ^{111}In-labeled antibody. The first patient studied received a 0.5 mg dose, the next patients received 1 mg dose, and five patients each received 2, 5, and 10 mg of antibody. The antibody was suspended in 200 ml of normal saline and administered over two hours. Vital signs were monitored at half-hour intervals during and for two hours following the infusion. Each patient was studied once. Following infusion, total body imaging, and in some cases, selected photon tomography were performed using a longitudinal tomographic imager. Scans were performed at 5, 24, 48, 72, and 144 hours post infusion. Plasma for pharmacological studies was obtained after one hour of infusion and at 0, 1, 5, 10, 30, and 60 minutes. Additional samples were drawn at 2, 3, 6, 24, and 48 hours post infusion. Urine was also collected over 48 hours to measure isotope excretion.

Measurement of Circulating Melanoma Antigen

Prior to study, individual serum samples were collected and sent to Hybritech, Inc. for measurement of P-97 melanoma antigen. Two hundred microliters of patient or normal serum was incubated for four hours with polystyrene beads bound to saturating doses of P-96.5. After incubation, the beads were washed and resuspended in 200 μl of 4% albumin in PBS solution, which contained 10 ng of a second antibody, P-8.2, which had been radiolabeled with iodine 125. P-8.2 recognizes a second epitope found on the surface of P-97 antigen. The beads were then incubated overnight, washed three times, and counted on a gamma counter. The results were calculated by comparing them to known quantities of antigen secreted from a ST-MEL cell line.

Measurement of Specific Binding of P-96.5 Monoclonal Antibody to Fresh Tumor Tissue In Vitro

The P-96.5 antibody was diluted in 0.01 M PBS containing 0.1% gelatin. One to three drops of antibody solution was added to cryostat tissue sections which were cut in 5 μm thicknesses, air dried, and fixed with acetone. The slide was then incubated for 30 to 60 minutes at room temperature in a moist chamber. It was rinsed with 0.1M PBS containing 0.01% thimerosal (PBST) for five minutes in a coplin jar, and excess buffer was filtered off. From one to three drops of a goat antimouse IgG-horseradish perioxidase-conjugated antibody (Cappel Laboratories, Cochranville, PA) was added, and the slide was incubated for 30 minutes at room temperature. After rinsing in PBS, three drops of a substrate solution containing 2 ml of ascetate buffer, two drops of acetate buffer, two drops of stock indicator solution, and one drop of 3% H_2O_2 was added and incubated for 20 mintues at room temperature. The slide was then rinsed with distilled water and counterstained for five minutes with Mayer's hematoxylin. The slide was rinsed with tap water and a cover slip was added along with 80% glycerol gelatin. The slide was examined for peroxidase stain by light microscopy.

146

RESULTS

Tumor Sites Imaged

The number and the precentage of sites imaged in relation to P-96.5 antibody dose are shown in Table 1. Of a total of 41 tumor sites that had been previously diagnosed by conventional x-rays, CT and radionucleide scans, 23 were visualized, for a true positive imaging rate of 56%. Eighteen previously documented metastatic sites did not visualize for a false negative rate of 44%. In no instance was imaging observed in metastatic sites that had not been previously confirmed. As the actual amount of antibody was increased, there was a definite dose-response effect noted. For example, only two out of nine metastatic sites (23%) were imaged at the 1 mg dose, in constrast to 11 out of 13 metastatic sites at the 10 mg dose (86%). In patients receiving a lower dose, there appeared to be a greater uptake of radiolabeled antibody in soft tissue sites of metastasis such as lung and lymph nodes, with lesser uptake observed in visceral areas, such as brain, liver, and bone. However, this was probably a reflection of the antibody dose administered, since several patients studied at the 10 mg dose had uptake in all known tumor sites. Optimal tumor imaging occurred from 72 to 144 hours post infusion.

During the entire follow-up period on each patient, large amounts of antibody were seen in liver, spleen, marrow, and lung, presumably in the vasculature and related to the long serum half-life of the antibody (see below). All patients were skin tested. A positive reaction was defined as a greater than 5 mm erythema or induration. The results of skin testing, the circulating antigen titers, and surface antigen reactivity on selected patient biopsies are shown in Table 2. Only one patient had a positive reaction to antibody and this patient was excluded. Only two patients out of 20 had circulating antigen levels above the upper range for normals (2 ng/ml). Of the four patient biopsies studied, three reacted with P-96.5 in vitro and two of these imaged in vivo.

Table 1
Radioimmunolocalization of Melanoma with ^{111}In-Labeled Monoclonal Antibody to P-97

Dose mg Ab	Patients	Known	Imaged (%)	Previously Unknown
0.5–1.0	5	10	2 (20)	0
2.0	5	8	5 (62)	0
5.0	5	10	5 (50)	0
10.0	5	13	11 (85)	0
Total	20	41	23 (56)	0

Toxicity

No clinical toxicity was noted. There were no significant changes in any laboratory parameters and no side effects (Table 3).

Pharmacology

Plasma samples were measured for clearance of the ^{111}In label by gamma counting. The clearance of the radioactive isotope from the plasma closely fit a one-compartmental open mathematical model. The mean plasma half-life in the patients was 40.7 hours. The total area under the plasma concentration curve (C × T) was 766.8 Ci/ml × minutes (Figure 1). The urinary excretion of the ^{111}In label is shown in Figure 2. Only 15% of the total dose of indium administered was eventually excreted. More rapid excretion occurred in the first six hours after the antibody infusion. It is not known from these studies whether the intact antibody or actual antibody fragments were present.

A summary of the pharmacologic data on the first 12 patients is shown in Table 4. The mean plasma $t_{1/2}$ appeared to be independent of the total dose of antibody administered. The distribution volume (Vd) decreased with an increasing dose of cold antibody. The percentage of the indium label excreted, however was unaffected by antibody dose. There was not

Table 2
Immunologic Parameters

No. Patients with + Skin Test to P-96.5 (0.1 μg)*	No. Patients with Elevated Serum Antigen P-97 (N = 1–2 ng/ml)†	No. Patients with Tumor Reactive with P-96.5 in Vitro
1/20	2/20	2/4‡

*Positive (+) test = 5 mm diameter erythema or induration.
†P-97 was found in serum of only 2 of 20 patients at > 2 ng/ml.
‡Of the 4 patients who reacted in vitro, only 2 of the 4 imaged.

Table 3
Toxicity Data: P-97 Monoclonal Ab[32]

Parameter	Prestudy	Post Inf:1 Day	Post Inf:7 Day
WBC (× 10³)	8.9 ± 4.7	8.5 ± 4.1	6.3 ± 2.1
HCT	39 ± 5.6	38.2 ± 6.1	36.8 ± 5.2
Platelet count (× 10³)	307 ± 147	333 ± 128	326 ± 136
SGOT	20.1 ± 9.1	18.6 ± 9.2	22.6 ± 12.4
BUN	14.3 ± 4.8	12.8 ± 4.7	11.3 ± 3.4
Creatinine	1.0 ± .17	1.0 ± .25	.94 ± .28
LDH	287 ± 141	233 ± 132	303 ± 143

148

a strong correlation between whether or not imaging occurred in the patient and the clearance of antibody from the plasma.

Following antibody administration, considerable nonspecific uptake of isotope in the liver, spleen, and bone marrow was observed. Disappearance of radioactivity in these organs was gradual, with considerable activity still present at 72 hours. Optimum visualization of tumor sites occurred at 72 and 144 hours.

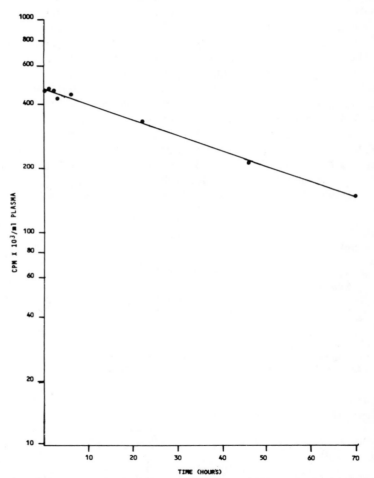

Figure 1 Typical plasma disappearance curve of the ^{111}In label from a patient who received 10 mg of mouse monoclonal antibody bearing a total of 2.5 μCi of 11 In label. For all patients studied and at all dose levels, plasma disappearance curves closely fit ($r^2 > 0.90$), a one compartment mathematical model for clearance.

Patient Examples

Representative examples of tumor imaging in two patients are shown in Figures 3 and 4. Case 1 is a 27-year-old white male with metastases to lung, duodenum, the left adrenal, cerebellum, skin, and pancreatic lymph nodes. He was scanned following administration of 10 mg of antibody. Spot views of his chest and abdominal area at 144 hours post infusion of antibody are shown. There was increased uptake of indium label in many of the areas mentioned, most particularly, in the large skin tumors

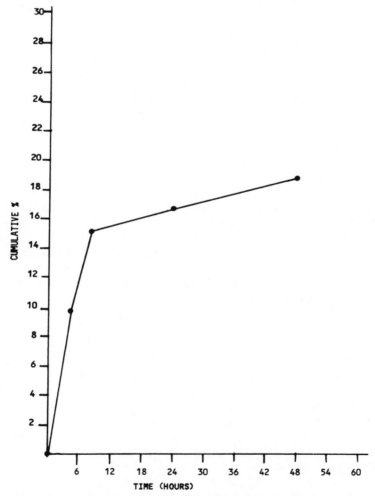

Figure 2 Typical urinary excretion curve of the ^{111}In label. In all patients, no more than 27% of the radiolabel was excreted over the two-day study period. Most of the radiolabel was excreted within the first six hours after administration.

Table 4
Melanoma Monoclonal Antibody Pharmacokinetics Summary

Patient No.	Total Dose (mg)	$t_{\frac{1}{2}}$ (min)	Vd (1)	C × T (μCi/ml × min)	Cumulative % Excreted (48 hrs)
1	1	639.5	8.6	117.4	19.3
2	1	833	8.5	155.9	36.1
3	1	2959	8.1	576.0	15.6
4	1	2110	5.8	576.0	19.1
	X̄	1653 ± 548	7.78 ± 0.66	656 ± 127	22.5 ± 4.6
5	2	1740	7.3	356	19.7
6	2	2415	6.2	470	28.4
7	2	2437	7.7	464	20.4
8	2	2287	6.3	560	18.0
9	2	1827	9.7	291	7.8
	X̄	2141 ± 149	7.5 ± 0.65	428 ± 47	18.9 ± 3.3
10	5	2037	5.0	579	12.1
11	5	2083	3.9	699	17.1
12	5	2443	4.2	767	18.8
	X̄	2188 ± 128	4.4 ± 0.3	682 ± 55	16.0 ± 2.0

seen in the left supraclavicular and the right inguinal area (arrows). Increased radioactivity was seen additionally in the spine as well as in the midabdominal area corresponding to the duodenal metastases. The second patient, Figure 4, is a 37-year-old white male who presented with masses in the mediastinum and in the right supraclavicular are; he received 5 mg of antibody. Tumor uptake was seen, despite the fact that the patient had recently received radiation therapy to the mediastinum.

DISCUSSION

We have tested 20 patients with malignant melanoma with escalating doses of ^{111}In-labeled monoclonal antibody (P-96.5). No toxicity was seen. Of the 41 previously diagnosed metastatic sites, a total of 23 imaged, the majority at antibody doses of 5 and 10 mg. The mean plasma half-life of ^{111}In was 40.7 hours and urinary excretion of isotope accounted for only 16% of the administered dose. Consistent with the long plasma half-time, significant uptake of isotope was seen in liver and spleen and marrow. Because of this increased non-specific uptake, optimum tumor imaging was noted from 72 to 144 hours following infusion.

The most noteworthy finding in this study was that improved imaging was seen following increasing doses of antibody while the specific activity of ^{111}In remained constant. The reason for this observation is

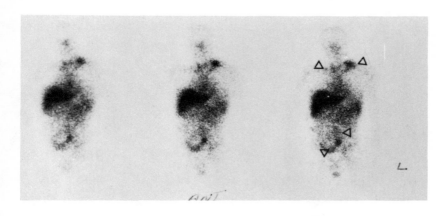

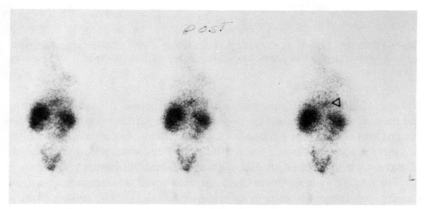

Figure 3 Selected images of a patient studied following 10 mg of P-96.5 at 144 hours. Increased uptake was noted in the right and left supraclavicular areas, the right pelvic area, abdomen and spine (arrows). There was still considerable background radioactivity in the liver and spleen even at 144 hours.

unknown. One possibility is that increasing amounts of cold antibody could rapidly block receptor sites in highly vascular organs such as the liver and spleen, with a gradually increased uptake of radiolabeled antibody in the tumor tissue as more of these sits were filled. Since P-96.5 is of the IgG 2A subclass, it could conceivably be bound by macrophage Fc receptors in these organs.[7] Alternatively, the antibody may bind to other normal tissues that express low concentration of the P-97 antigen,[8] thereby allowing more uptake of radiolabled antibody at high affinity tumor sites.

The pharmacology of the ^{111}In-labeled antibody is quite similar to that described using a ^{111}In-labeled anti-CEA antibody in the nude mouse.[9] Unlike iridium 131 coupled to monoclonal antibody, ^{111}In-coupled antibody is quite stable in vivo with little loss of bound isotope.

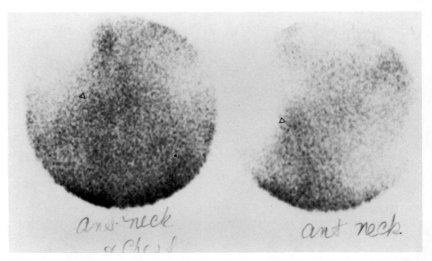

Figure 4 Patient 2. Increased uptake noted in the right supraclavicular and anterior cervical areas (arrows) as previously documented clinically. Antibody dose was 5 mg.

Uptake of isotope in tumor tissue gradually increased over 72 hours in the mouse model. Because of its stability, very little ^{111}In-label was excreted, and the ratio of isotope in tumor to that of other tissues was high enough for adequate imaging without background subtraction procedures, as have been utilized in studies with polyclonal antibodies.[1,2]

Surprisingly, few patients had elevated levels of circulating antigen despite high tumor burdens in several individuals. It is unknown at present whether low antigen levels are related to circulating immune complexes or decreased antigen shedding by tumor. The data on immunoperoxidase staining of tumor tissue are too preliminary to draw conclusions as to whether any correlation exists between in vivo imaging and in vitro positivity for P-97.

Although these preliminary results are encouraging, further studies are needed to define the optimum dose and administration of antibody and isotope, as well as studies to determine the optimum methods for radioimaging.

REFERENCES

1. Goldenberg DM, DeLand F, Kim E, et al: Use of radiolabeled antibodies to carcinoembryonic antigen for the detection and localization of diverse cancers by external photoscanning. *N Engl J Med* 1978;298:1384–1388
2. Mach JP, Carrell S, Merenda C, et al: In vivo localization of anti-CEA antibody to colon carcinoma. Can the results obtained in the nude mice model be extrapolated to the patient situation? *Eur J Cancer* 1978;113–120.

3. Brown JP, Nishiyama K, Hellstrom I, et al: Structural characterization of human melanoma-associated antigen P-97 with monoclonal antibodies. *J Immunol* 1981;237:539–546.
4. Brown JP, Woodbury RG, Hart CE, et al: Quantitative analysis of melanoma-associated antigen P-97 in normal and neoplastic tissues. *Proc Natl Acad Sci USA* 1981;78:539–543.
5. Woodbury RG, Brown JP, Yeh M-Y, et al: Identification of a cell surface protein, P-97, in human melanomas and certain other neoplasms. *Proc Natl Acad Sci USA* 1980;77:2183–2186.
6. Hellstrom I, Brown JP, Hellstrom KE: Monoclonal antibodies to two determinants of melanoma-antigen P-97 act synergistically in complement dependent cytotoxicity. *J Immunol* 1981;127(1):157–160.
7. Steplewski Z, Lubeck MD, Koprowski H: Human macrophages armed with murine immunoglobulin G2a antibodies to tumor destroy human cancer cells. *Science* 1983;221:865–867.
8. Woodbury RG, Brown JP, Loop SM, et al: Analysis of normal neoplastic human tissues for the tumor-associated protein P-97. *Int J Cancer* 1981;27:145–149.
9. Stern P, Hagan P, Halpern S, et al: The effect of the radiolabel on the kinetics of monoclonal anti-CEA in a nude mouse-human colon tumor model, in Mitchell MS, Oettgen HF, (eds): *Progress in Cancer Research and Therapy, Hybridomas in Cancer Diagnosis and Treatment.* New York, Raven Press, 1982, vol 21, pp 245–253.

17   *Monoclonal Antibodies to Human Prostate Tissue**

R.H. Raynor, T. Mohanakumar,
C.W. Monclure, T.A. Hazra

Carcinoma of the prostate is the most common form of genitourinary cancer and accounts for about 17% of all cancers in males. Little is understood about the epidemiology of this cancer, other than the facts that the age gradient for the disease after age 50 is steeper than for any other cancer type, and that the incidence in black males has strikingly increased in the last several decades. Therapy is often effective when aimed at prostate cancers in early stages of their development; however, the characteristics of this malignancy are such that detection is sometimes difficult, and in many cases the disease is well advanced with metastatic lesions formed prior to diagnosis. Therefore, with respect to prostate cancer, there is a need for early detection methods as well as for novel therapeutic approaches and more effective means to monitor the course of the disease. It is well established that tumor cells can express new antigens as a result of malignant transformation and may lose normal membrane antigens as well. Antigenic changes are often important clinically because they may reflect a state of differentiation not always detectable by standard morphological criteria. In the present study, we have developed a series of monoclonal antibodies to cell surface antigens of the prostate carcinoma cell lines, PC-3[1] and DU-145.[2] Preliminary characterization of these antibodies indicates varying degrees of specificity for malignant prostate epithelium, and one antibody, KR-P8, detects a unique prostate-specific marker that has been previously undescribed.

MATERIALS AND METHODS

Antisera

Fluorescein isothiocyanate (FITC)-conjugated goat anti-mouse IgG, was purchased from Cappel Laboratories (Cochranville, PA).

---

*Accepted in principle.

Cell Lines

PC-3[1] was derived from a prostatic bone metastasis and the DU-145 line[2] was derived from a brain metastasis. Both lines were cultured in RPMI 1640 medium supplemented with 7% fetal calf serum (FCS), 2 mM L-glutamine, 100 μg/ml penicillin and 100 μg/ml streptomycin (all from GIBCO, Grand Island, NY).

Animals

Female BALB/c mice (15–20 g) were purchased from Charles River Laboratories (Wilmington, MA). All animals were housed in laminar flow isolation cabinets (Contamination Control, Inc., Landsdale, PA) within the animal resources facilities of the Medical College of Virginia.

Human Tissues

Portions of human prostates were obtained from Dr. T.I. Malinin through the National Prostatic Cancer Project (NIH Grant, #CA 15480). Tissues were designated as normal prostate, BPH, or prostatic carcinoma and were kept frozen at − 70C. Other tissues, including lung, liver, kidney, testis, colon, lymph node, and urinary bladder, were obtained from autopsy specimens.

Hybridoma Production

The monoclonal antibodies resulted from fusions of mouse myeloma cells, P3-NS1-Ag4-1, with spleen cells from BALB/c mice that had been immunized with cells of the PC-3 and/or DU-145 cell lines. Spleen cells were fused with the myeloma cells at a ratio of two spleen cells to one myeloma cell in the presence of polyethyleneglycol 6000 (Sigma, St. Louis, MO) according to the procedure of Kennett.[3] Ultimately, the hybridomas were grown in HB 101 medium (Hana Biologics, Inc., Berkeley, CA), which was supplemented with 1% Hy-Clone FCS (Sterile Systems, Inc., Logan, UT), sodium pyruvate (1 mM), L-glutamine, and penicillin/streptomycin. The supernatants from these cultures were used as the source of antibodies for all assays.

Immunofluorescence Assay

Cell-surface reactivity of the antibodies was judged by indirect immunofluorescence assays, whereby 100 μl of culture supernatant was incubated with 1×10^5 cells for 30 minutes at 40C. After three washes with IF wash medium (RPMI 1640 containing 10% FCS and 0.1% sodium azide), the cells were stained with 50 μl of a 1:50 dilution of FITC-conjugated goat anti-mouse IgG and examined for fluorescence using a Leitz Ortho-Lux II fluorescence microscope equipped with epi-illumination. Cells stained with HB 101 culture supernatants from the NS-1 myeloma cell line served as the negative control.

Immunoperoxidase Assays

Normal neoplastic tissue sections were tested for reactivity with KR-P8 by immunoperoxidase assays. Both frozen sections and fixed paraffin-embedded sections were used. Paraffin-embedded sections were deparaffinized by soaking the slides in two changes of xylene for one hour each and rehydrated by treatment with graded alcohols (15 minutes each in 100%, 95% and 90% ethanol) and overnight with distilled water. Antibody reactivity was tested using the Vectastain ABC kit for mouse IgG (Vector Laboratories, Burlington, CA). Sections were counterstained with Gill's hemotoxylin (Fisher Scientific, Pittsburg, PA), dehydrated in graded alcohols and mounted with Permount (Fisher Scientific). Controls for all tissues consisted of staining serial sections with HB 101 supernatants from NS-1 myelomas. Sections treated in this manner gave no detectable background reactivity.

RESULTS

Monoclonal antibodies were prepared to components on the surface of cells of the carcinoma cell lines PC-3 and DU-145 as described in the materials and methods. As a result of these procedures, we have produced six stable hybridomas that secrete antibodies recognizing determinants present on the prostate cell lines, and that demonstrate varying degrees of prostate specificity as well. These antibodies are described in Table 1. As shown,

Table 1
Monoclonal Antibody Reactivity Patterns

Designation	Immunizing Cells	Antibody Subclass* Secreted	Immunofluorescence† Reactivity		
			DU-145	PC-3	T-24
I KR–P1	DU145/PC3	IgG$_1$	+	+	+
KR–P4	PC3	IgG$_1$	+	+	+
II KR–P2	DU145/PC3	IgG$_{2b}$	+	+	−
KR–P8	PC3	IgG$_1$	+	+	−
III KR–P3	DU145/PC3	IgG$_{2a}$	−	+	−
KR–P5	PC3	IgG$_1$	−	+	−

*Determined by Ouchterlony analysis.
†Antibody reactivity was judged by indirect immunofluorescence as described in the materials and methods.

158

some mice were immunized with a mixture of the two prostate cell lines while others immunized with only one line. The subclass of antibody secreted by each hybridoma was determined by Ouchterlony analysis. Antibody reactivity with each of the two prostate lines and to one bladder carcinoma cell line (T-24) was tested by indirect immunofluorescence assays. The reason for testing reactivity with the bladder line was based on reports of antigen similarity between these two tissue types. Interestingly, the antibody reactivity patterns fell into three groups. Two antibodies (KR-P1 and KR-P4) reacted with all three lines. Two KR-P3 and KR-P8) reacted only with the prostate lines detecting antigens common to both lines, and KR-P3 and KR-P5 reacted only with the PC-3 line. Such reactivity profiles indicate antigenic heterogeneity among the two prostate cell lines that are isolated from the different metastatic lesions.

To further establish the specificity of the antibodies, we next tested the antibodies for reactivity against a number of malignant and normal cell lines. As judged by indirect immunofluorescence, none of the cell lines listed in Table 2, including one cytomegalovirus (CMV) infected fibroblast line were found to be reactive with any of the antibodies.

More extensive tests of tissue reactivity have been conducted with one of the antibodies, KR-P8. As shown in Table 3, although KR-P8 was originally prepared against a malignant prostate cell line, the antigen recognized by this antibody was found on benign hypertrophic and normal prostate tissue samples.

The antigen was detected on unfixed, frozen sections of tissues as well as on formalin-fixed, paraffin-embedded sections of prostate, indicating that the antigen is stable to routine histological fixation procedures. The pattern of reactivity of KR-P8 as shown here is restricted to prostate based on the absence of reactivity with sections of tissue removed from the bladder, kidney, liver, colon, testis and lung (Table 3). The antibody also demonstrated reactivity with one lymph node specimen that was judged to be positive for prostate metastasis upon subsequent

Table 2
Cell Lines *Not* Reacting with Antiprostate
Monoclonal Antibodies*

Designation	Source
BL	Pheochromocytoma
AD	Melanoma
MCF-7	Breast carcinoma
MDA-MB-231	Breat carcinoma
SKNSH	Neuroblastoma
ES	Normal fibroblast
Townes-MRC5	CMV-infected fibroblast

*Reactivity of the cell line was judged by indirect immunofluorescence assays.

Table 3
Profile of KR-P8 Tissue Reactivity

Tissue	KR-P8 Reactivity*
Prostate	
Normal	+ (see Figure 2)
BPH	+
Carcinoma	+
Urinary bladder	−
Kidney	−
Liver	−
Colon	−
Testis	−
Lung	−

*Sections of tissue were stained with KR-P8 and developed using the Vectastain ABC kit as described in the materials and methods.

histological examination (data not shown). On all of 15 prostate specimens (eight carcinoma, three BPH and four normal) reactivity of KR-P8 was evident within the glandular epithelium of the prostate. This is demonstrated by the staining pattern shown in Figure 1 (A and B). The connective tissue, smooth-muscle stroma of the prostate is free of reactivity with KR-P8. The KR-P8 antigen was found to be present within the cytoplasm of the epithelial cells and, in more concentrated form, on the luminal surfaces of these cells. This pattern of reactivity indicates that the antigen recognized by KR-P8 is a product that is secreted by the glandular cells. This is supported by the fact that antibody reactivity is also seen within the amorphous material that accumulates within some of the glands.

Further studies have shown that the KR-P8 antigen is distinct from prostatic acid phosphatase and is also different from the recently described prostate-specific antigen (data not shown).

DISCUSSION

This report describes the initial characterization of a panel of monoclonal antibodies that show varying degrees of specificity for prostate tissue. As shown in Table 1, differential reactivity patterns verify the existence of cell-surface antigenic heterogeneity between the two prostate cell lines, PC-3 and DU-145. In addition, further studies with the KR-P8 monoclonal antibody indicate that this antibody detects a unique prostate specific marker. The KR-P8 antigen is present on all sections of prostate tested, including normal, BPH and malignant specimens, but is absent from a variety of other tissue types (Table 3). This antigen has furthermore been shown to be distinct from the previously reported and well-characterized prostatic acid phosphatase[4] and prostate specific antigen.[5]

The KR-P8 antigen is stable to routine histological fixation procedures, and the antibody demonstrates potential as a diagnostic agent for identification of prostate as the primary source of distant metastases.

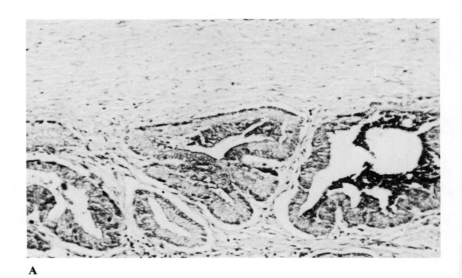

A

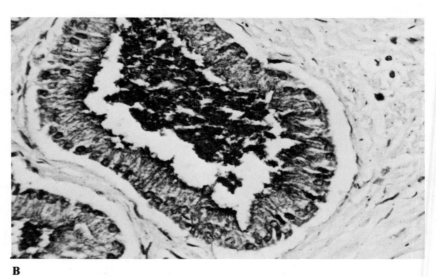

B

Figure 1 Detection of KR-P8 antigen in sections of normal human prostate. Paraffin sections of normal prostate were stained with KR-P8 and developed using the Vectastain ABC kit. Sections were counterstained with hematoxylin (**A** = $50 \times$; **B** = $125 \times$).

The therapeutic potential of this antibody is now being tested in the nude mouse model by its ability to home to and bind a growing, subcutaneously implanted human prostate tumor.

REFERENCES

1. Kaighn ME, Narauam KS, Ohnuki Y, et al: *Invest Urol* 1979;17:16–23.
2. Mickey DD, Stone KR, Wunderli H, et al: in Murphy GP (ed): *Models for Prostate Cancer*. New York, Alan R. Liss, Inc., 1980;67–84.
3. Kennett RH, et al (eds): *Monoclonal Antibodies: Hybridomas. A New Dimension in Biological Analyses*. New York, Plenum Press, 1980, 365.
4. Gutman AB, Gutman EB: *J Clin Invest* 1983;17:473–478.
5. Nadji M, Tabei SZ, Castro A, et al: *Cancer* 1981;48:1229–1232.

Closing Remarks

We have heard a series of interesting papers regarding the use of monoclonal antibodies in the diagnosis, localization and treatment of malignancy. It is clear that there are many obstacles to these in vivo applications of monoclonal antibodies. Some of these were anticipated, such as antigenic modulation, selection for antigen-negative cells or a host response to foreign immunoglobulin. Others were less expected, such as a limited host capability to clear antibody-coated cells, or the shedding of cell-surface antigens into the circulation.

These are some of the problems that face us, but it is encouraging to see how far the field has advanced. The discovery of monoclonal antibodies has been a major factor in reviving the hope that immunopotentiation will be useful in the treatment of malignancy. Monoclonal antibodies have allowed the definition by phenotype of cell subsets, previously unknown, that function in host defense. The ability to derive monoclonal antibodies against tumors, and the use of these antibodies to potentiate tumor killing, has obviated the criticism that spontaneous malignancies may not be immunogenic and consequently not subject to immune rejection. The use of monoclonal antibodies has revived the search for tumor-specific antigens with a precision not previously possible. Results such as those presented here suggest that even if tumor antigens are rarely unique — are expressed on some other tissues or at some other point of development — they may nonetheless have sufficient specificity to greatly enhance the selectivity of treatment. The best candidate for a truly tumor-specific antigen is immunoglobulin idiotype and, as Dr. Miller reviewed for us, the use of monoclonal antibodies against idiotypes on B-cell lymphomas has provided the most encouraging results to date for the use of monoclonal antibodies in tumor therapy.

Despite these advances, we are still relatively ignorant about the in vivo effects of antibodies against tumor targets. From studies such as those by Dr. Steplewski and others, we know that the effectiveness of cell destruction is dependent on the antibody subclass and on the nature of the target antigen. Cell killing is mediated by host cells, probably fixed macrophages within the lymphoid organs, particularly the liver and spleen. Although conjugation of antibodies with toxic compounds may increase the toxicity of the antibody itself, an important area for further research is the examination of the mechanisms by which monoclonal antibodies against cell surface antigens interact with host defense mechanisms to destroy the target cells. The greatest hope for destroying tumor cells by

164

the use of anti-tumor antibodies lies in the activation of the host to destroy the tumors. Simply on the basis of numbers, it is unlikely that the antibody alone, no matter how toxic, can destroy tumors with sufficient specificity and efficiency to constitute successful therapy. We therefore need to know more about how antibody-coated targets are destroyed. This will require an expansion of studies in animals. These will be facilitated by the fact that monoclonal antibodies have allowed the definition, in both primates and mice, of molecular homologues of human cell-surface antigens.

The definition of cell-surface antigens on normal cells by monoclonal antibodies, and the ability to isolate the antigens has allowed investigators to define the function of many of these cell "markers." It is clear that most, if not all, surface antigens are there for a purpose. This is likely to be of considerable importance with regard to the in vivo effects of antibodies against cell-surface antigens, especially if the antibodies either amplify or block the normal activity of the target antigen. For example, antibodies against the "T3" antigen are mitogenic for $T3^+$ cells and it seems likely that this may relate to the systemic side effects of this antibody that have been reviewed here. Similarly, Dr. Drew noted that treatment of a pancreatic carcinoma with a (relatively) tumor specific antibody produced profound diarrhea without an increase in amylase. This is conceivably due to the release of an agent such as vasoactive intestinal peptide from target cells.

Regardless of whether those serve as examples, it is clear that antibodies can alter cell function, as well as cell location or viability. Monoclonal antilymphocyte antibodies, therefore, may even subserve the function of certain lymphokines in altering host defense. It seems likely that effects of antibodies on target-cell function will be a significant area for future research.

I look forward to future meetings such as this. Despite the obstacles that have been presented, the future appears promising.

William E. Seaman

Index

170

172

174